D1124453

# LAW & ETHICS
## IN DIAGNOSTIC IMAGING
### A N D
## THERAPEUTIC  RADIOLOGY

# LAW & ETHICS
## IN DIAGNOSTIC IMAGING
### A N D
## THERAPEUTIC RADIOLOGY
### WITH RISK MANAGEMENT
### AND SAFETY APPLICATIONS

A n n   M .   O b e r g f e l l ,   J D ,   R T ( R )

**Associate Professor**
**Clinical Education Coordinator**
Radiologic Technology Program
University of Louisville
Louisville, Kentucky

SAUNDERS
*An Imprint of Elsevier*

SAUNDERS
*An Imprint of Elsevier*
The Curtis Center
Independence Square West
Philadelphia, PA 19106

**Library of Congress Cataloging-in-Publication Data**

Law and ethics in diagnostic imaging & therapeutic radiology : with risk management and safety applications / [edited by] Ann M. Obergfell. — 1st ed.
     p.  cm.
   ISBN-13: 978-0-7216-5062-3          ISBN-10: 0-7216-5062-7
     1. Radiologists—Malpractice—United States.  2. Diagnostic Imaging—United States.  3. Radiotherapy—United States.  4. Medical ethics—United States.  I. Obergfell, Ann M.
     [DNLM: 1. Diagnostic Imaging—United States.  2. Radiotherapy. 3. Jurisprudence.  4. Ethics, Medi.  WN 33 AA1 L4 1995]
   KF2910.R333L39    1995
   346.7303'32—dc20
   [347.306332]
   DNLM/DLC                                              95–10278

LAW & ETHICS

Copyright © 1995 by Saunders

All rights reserved. No part of this publication may be reproduced or transmitted in any form or by any means, electronic or mechanical, including photocopy, recording, or any information storage and retrieval system, without permission in writing from the publisher.

Permissions may be sought directly from Elsevier's Health Sciences Rights Department in Philadelphia, PA, USA: phone: (+1) 215 239 3804, fax: (+1) 215 239 3805, e-mail: healthpermissions@elsevier.com. You may also complete your request on-line via the Elsevier homepage (http://www.elsevier.com), by selecting 'Customer Support' and then 'Obtaining Permissions'.

ISBN-13: 978-0-7216-5062-3
ISBN-10: 0-7216-5062-7

Printed in United States of America

Last digit is the print number:   9   8

TO

My Parents

David and Luanne Obergfell

Who gave me a strong foundation on which to build

# P R E F A C E

Can I lose my job if I refuse to do a procedure? What can happen to me if I blow the whistle on unethical or illegal behavior in my workplace? What should I do if I'm asked to do something that I'm not qualified to do? What and how much should I document concerning diagnostic procedures? What are the patient's rights? These and many other questions are the kind I am asked as I travel around the country speaking on law and ethics in the radiologic sciences.

In an attempt to answer some of these questions and to explain the relationship between diagnostic imaging and therapeutic science and the law, I have organized a text that is an introduction to law and ethics as well as risk management and safety. The contributing authors all have special expertise in the areas in which they have written and all practice in the fields of law, risk management, or education.

The book is intended to be an overview and to offer information in the following areas: ethics, with special emphasis on the Code of Ethics; the law; civil law; medical negligence; documentation, patient's rights, and informed consent; employment law; labor law; risk management; safety; equipment safety; whistle blowing; and education. Applications in the day-to-day practice of the radiologic sciences have been utilized to explain some of the topics covered. The book is designed to be used as a text book for the classroom and a reference book for the department or facility.

Sample forms for documentation, consent, and competency evaluation have been included in the text. The reader is encouraged to review these forms and to adapt them to the specific health care setting. It is important to remember, however, that any forms adopted by a facility should be reviewed by risk management and legal counsel to make sure that they meet the needs of the facility and comply with specific legal and regulatory requirements of the jurisdiction (i.e., state or province).

The reader will gain a basic understanding of important issues affecting health care and the role of the technologist or therapist. Liability related to practice in the radiologic sciences is reviewed. However, since laws applying to the delivery of health care services vary from state to state and may change as case law develops and statutes and regulations are enacted, individuals seeking legal opinion should not use this text as a legal treatise, but should consult local counsel.

Every attempt has been made to locate and correct errors in the text; however, some errors may have gone undetected. If you locate errors or have constructive comments concerning the text, I would like to hear from you.

It is my hope that this text will assist radiologic science professionals in understanding the importance of the work performed in imaging and therapy departments and help focus their practice through strong ethical, legal, and educational principles in such a way that it benefits the patient, the technologist, the institution, and the profession.

Ann M. Obergfell, JD, RT(R)

# A C K N O W L E D G M E N T S

No endeavor is complete until you acknowledge and thank those individuals who made the work possible. The following people have given their assistance and support and to them I am eternally grateful.

- My program Director, Frances Campeau, the interim director of Allied Health, Dr. Patricia Walker, and the interim Dean of the College of Health and Social Services, Dr. Richard Swigart, all of whom supported me during the course of this project.
- My faculty colleagues, Dr. Mike Connor, Mike Goode, Don Pack, and Mark Crosthwaite, who helped pick up the slack.
- My contributing authors Angeline, Cathy, Mark, Randy, Ruby, and Tom, without whose efforts and expertise this book would not be possible.
- Michael Bloyd, Betty Clark, LaMont Coverstone, and Becky Zeller, who helped gather information for the text and the appendices.
- Sophia Fleming, who had to decipher the legalese before she could type and edit.
- Lisa Biello and the staff at W. B. Saunders, who gave able assistance to this rookie writer and editor.
- The students in the Radiography Program at the University of Louisville, who inspire and challenge me every day.
- And to my legal and radiologic science friends, who have taught me that the worlds of law and medicine can exist side by side.

Ann M. Obergfell, JD, RT(R)

# K E Y   T O   C I T A T I O N S

The endnotes on several of the chapters use legal citations that vary from the traditional cites found in medical or health related journals.

The citation system utilizes a series of numbers and letters to identify where the reader can locate the specific case or law. A sample of such a citation is:

**78 SW2d 478**

The number 78 indicates the volume of the reporter series in which the case is found. The letters SW2d indicate the Southwestern Reporter 2nd Series. The final number indicates the page in the volume where the case starts or the specific language cited is located.

The following reporters, codes, or reports are found in the text:

| | |
|---|---|
| **CFR** | **Code of Federal Regulations** |
| **FEP** | **Fair Employment Practices** |
| **F2d** | **Federal Reporter Second Series** |
| **FSupp** | **Federal Supplement** |
| **NW2d** | **Northwest Reporter Second Series** |
| **NYS2d** | **New York Supplement Second Series** |
| **P2d** | **Pacific Reporter Second Series** |
| **So2d** | **Southern Reporter Second Series** |
| **SCt** | **Supreme Court Reporter** |
| **US** | **United States Reporter** |
| **USC** | **United States Code** |
| **USCA** | **United States Codes Annotated** |

Reporter series for the particular state can generally be found in a public library. Reporters and codes for other jurisdictions can be found in a law library. Law libraries are usually associated with a local court house or hall of justice. The local Bar Association will be able to give the reader information on law library resources.

# C O N T R I B U T O R S

## CATHY K. AVDEVICH, MEd, RT(R)
Lecturer, School of Education
University of Louisville
Louisville, KY
■ CHAPTERS 10, 11, 12

## RUBY D. FENTON, JD
Attorney at Law
Rogers, Fuller, and Pitt
Louisville, KY
■ CHAPTER 13

## J. THOMAS GALLE, JD
Attorney at Law
Louisville, KY
■ CHAPTER 5

## ANGELINE GOLDEN, JD
Appellate Attorney—Special Fund
Labor Cabinet
Division of Special Fund
Louisville, KY
■ CHAPTER 3

## ANN M. OBERGFELL, JD, RT(R)
Associate Professor
Clinical Education Coordinator
University of Louisville
Louisville, KY
■ CHAPTERS 1, 2, 6, 7, 14

## RAYMOND L. SMITH, JR., JD
Attorney at Law
Rogers, Fuller, and Pitt
Louisville, KY
■ CHAPTERS 8, 9

## MARK WEBSTER, JD
Attorney—Chief Ombudsman
Department of Workers Claims
Commonwealth of Kentucky
Frankfort, KY
■ CHAPTER 4

# C O N T E N T S

# 1

# Introduction

Ann M. Obergfell

Health care is constantly changing. From these changes flow many issues that affect diagnostic imaging and therapeutic science practitioners. A truly comprehensive overview of issues affecting these professions would fill volumes. However, a relatively concise review of these issues, with suggestions on methods to adopt or adapt for the clinical setting, can assist technologists, therapists, managers, and educators as they make their way through the minefield of change.

Ethics; law; standard of care and informed consent; documentation and record keeping; labor-management relations; employment; risk management; and safety are but a few of the topics affecting diagnostic imaging and therapeutic radiology.

## ETHICS

Many view ethics as a philosophical analysis of the way people ought to behave toward one another. In fact, ethics encompasses not only what ought to be done but also what must be done in an orderly and organized society.

Ethical considerations are not isolated in the ivory towers of academia but play an important role in both personal and professional life and in the day-to-day activities of health care delivery. Each person who participates in the delivery of care must consciously and unconsciously abide by ethical principles and standards.

The American Society of Radiologic Technologists (ASRT) has adopted a professional code of ethics for those who practice in the radiologic sciences. Those professionals who are registered by the American Registry of Radiologic Technologists (ARRT) sign a statement agreeing to abide by the enumerated principles of the ASRT Code of Ethics. Others who practice in the field are held to the same standards through legal and ethical theories and concepts.

## LAW

Medicine and law interact regularly to play an important role in the delivery of health care. The relationship between law and medicine provides a healthy system of checks and balances which can create a positive environment for anyone entering the system as a patient.

Health care professionals have an obligation to do no harm and a duty to provide reasonable care for the patient who seeks their assistance. Although these professionals are not expected to be perfect, they are expected to meet the standard of care established for their particular area of practice and always to consider the best interests of the patient.

When this system breaks down and a patient is injured or suffers some harm from the unreasonable actions of a health care provider, the law steps in to protect the patient's interests. Many in health care view this as an intrusion and vilify the legal profession for creating an adversarial environment, forcing the practice of "defensive" medicine, and driving up the cost of health care. While these points are debatable and statistics are used by both sides to prove their points, it is clear that, when the system works, the patient is the ultimate beneficiary. The quality of care will improve or, when it does not, the patient will be justly compensated.

Health care professionals may become part of the legal system as parties or as witnesses in medical negligence or malpractice litigation. Following an initial complaint, the second step of the process continues through discovery, which includes the taking of depositions and a thorough investigation of the incident. Upon completion of discovery, either the case will go to trial or the parties will make a settlement agreement. The legal process can be very time consuming; the entire process may take several years depending on the need for extensive discovery and on the rules of the jurisdiction.

## Civil Liability

The legal community is often asked to represent injured parties as they seek redress from the individual or organization that has allegedly harmed them. The injury suffered by the patient/plaintiff can come in the form of actual physical injury, emotional distress, or economic loss because of lost wages or employment opportunities. Legal claims of assault, battery, false imprisonment, and defamation could arise from improper or inadequate health care practices. In these cases, the legal system is asked to protect those who cannot protect themselves or to assist those who should be compensated for their injuries.

## Negligence

The most common legal principle used in an attempt to make the injured party whole is the concept of medical negligence. This theory requires that the injured party prove that a duty owed by the health care professional to a patient was breached and that, because of this breach, the patient was injured. The legal twists and turns are easy to follow when analyzed in terms of the professional obligation to patients and the liability that arises from failure to perform in a manner required by the profession and the law.

## STANDARD OF CARE AND INFORMED CONSENT

Through guidelines and education, the profession establishes a standard of care that sets parameters within which the professional is obligated to practice. The law does not expect the health care professional to perform miracles, but it does require that the practitioner meet the standard established by the profession.

The standard of care for diagnostic imaging and therapeutic science is established by the profession through its scope of practice and educational requirements. Curricula have been developed for the radiologic sciences to direct the education of future professionals and therefore establish a standard for those who practice or will practice in the various fields. The *legal standard* is defined as the degree of care and skill utilized by a reasonable professional practicing in the same or similar circumstances.

While the professions direct the practice, it is the patient who determines the type of care that is rendered after consultation with the physician or other health professional. Consenting to treatment requires that the patient be informed about the benefits, risks, and alternatives of the proposed procedure. Only after the patient has this information can a truly informed decision concerning medical care be made.

## DOCUMENTATION AND RECORD KEEPING

Documentation can be the health care professional's best friend or worst enemy. Although records are required by statute, regulation, and institutional policy, many legal claims are lost by the defendant health care provider because of a failure to keep accurate records concerning the care delivered and the progress made by the patient during the course of treatment.

Some jurisdictions are of the opinion that, if it wasn't written, it didn't happen. Memory will not serve the health care professional in a case in which a person was injured and no records or incomplete notes were kept.

Each jurisdiction has requirements for the type of records to be kept by an institution, as well as guidelines concerning how the records are to be maintained and for how long. Radiographs and other images are generally part of the record; as such, it is imperative that they be maintained properly and for the appropriate length of time. Departmental and clinical procedures and protocols should be drafted to follow the statutory criteria.

## LABOR-MANAGEMENT RELATIONS

Accurate record keeping and open communication are critical in the relationship between the patient and the health care provider. Likewise, precise record keeping, notice, and open, two-way communication are essential to a healthy association between employers and employees.

The service industry has been targeted for unionization, and in many areas of the country, unions have long been a part of the health care delivery system. If unions are present in a facility, it is critical that the management team recognize the relationship and act according to any existing agreements or contracts between the union and the facility. If unions are not part of the system, methods that may help the facility remain union free include open communication, fairness in employment practices, decent working conditions, and a relationship between employers and employees that nurtures a healthy and happy work environment.

## EMPLOYMENT ISSUES

While many labor problems center around the working conditions in a facility, other laws come into play which should, if followed correctly, create a positive work environment for both employer and employee. Laws affecting hiring practices, discrimination, harassment, and safety of patients and employees all play important roles in creating a quality work environment. Employers should be familiar with these laws and understand how the workplace is affected when they are violated.

Health care facilities, regardless of size, should draft policies that address employment concerns and must educate all employees about the organization's expectations regarding such issues. The employer must, if necessary, be prepared to investigate a complaint and discipline an employee—whether management or staff—if an employment policy has been violated.

## RISK MANAGEMENT

The role of risk management is to minimize risk and potential financial loss for the institution, as well as to protect the institution's good name. Hospitals have risk management departments that handle the entire institution, from grounds to intensive care unit. While the diagnostic imaging department is included within this umbrella coverage, it is important that a departmental risk management plan be developed. This plan will allow management and staff to work together to determine and minimize any risks associated with the department's activities.

Whether part of a larger institution or a freestanding clinic, every imaging or therapy department should institute risk management practices that help minimize the risks in the department or center. Tracking trends in the department, immediate and decisive response to incidents, and followup on policies will help the facility minimize financial loss associated with incidents or injuries.

## SAFETY

Equipment safety is but a small portion of all a facility's safety practices. Regulations and safety requirements in the workplace are abundant, and it is critical that managers and staff understand the policies affecting their work environment.

The safety of patients, employees, and visitors is part of the reasonable practice of any health care facility. Common problems, such as water spills and poor lighting, are as important as electrical and chemical hazards. All members of the health care delivery team must be aware of the safety risks associated with their facility and prepared to correct or report any problems that arise.

The radiologic science professions use the most sophisticated equipment available in health care today. The technologists and therapists who work with this equipment must be familiar with the operation and day-to-day maintenance of that equipment. The theory that radiologic science professionals need only know which buttons to push is inaccurate and inappropriate in light of the responsibilities placed on them by the standards of the profession and the regulations imposed by such administrative agencies as the Occupational Safety and Health Administration (OSHA) and the Environmental Protection Agency (EPA).

## WHISTLEBLOWING

Many problems in health care settings go undetected or unreported for long periods of time because employees are afraid to "blow the whistle." The fear of reporting may allow small problems to grow into major dilemmas for which the facility may be financially liable. The fear of retaliation, in the form of loss of employment or creation of a hostile work environment, prevents many workers from reporting problems to management or to outside investigatory agencies, such as OSHA, EPA, the Nuclear Regulatory Commission (NRC), or the Equal Employment Opportunity Commission (EEOC).

Federal regulations protect federal employees from retaliation for whistleblowing, and some states have adopted similar statutes for state employees. Other, nongovernment employees may be protected by public policy considerations and may have legal claims for retaliation or wrongful discharge if, after the complaint, a discriminatory employment practice occurs.

Employees may be required to follow their conscience when reporting inappropriate or dangerous practices. The law can protect them in some cases as long as both employer and employee have followed appropriate procedures.

## EDUCATION

The profession has also set educational standards. Accrediting bodies have been instituted to assess programs in all of the radiologic sciences with the hope of creating quality educational opportunities for students, technologists, and therapists. The many years of only on-the-job training and "rising through the ranks" are coming to an end. Health care delivery, particularly in the radiologic sciences, has become technologically sophisticated and increasingly complex.

The old educational philosophy of "see one, do one, teach one" no longer meets the needs of the patient or the profession; critical thinking has become the norm. Technologists and therapists must work with high-tech equipment and patients whose conditions warrant special care and consideration. Professionals must be able to adapt their practice to the special needs of the facility and the patient.

Hospital administration requires managers and supervisors to understand management principles and to run their departments efficiently and effectively, as managers. Educators must constantly adjust how and what they teach so that new technologies and procedures can be introduced to future radiologic science professionals.

Radiologic science professionals are required to maintain and improve their professional competencies. Legally, the standard of care requires that each professional remain current in the field in which he or she practices. Health care providers who are inactive and subsequently return to the field must be prepared to practice at the current level of technology, not that of the time when they went inactive or were in school.

## CONCLUSION

Health care delivery is a complex, technologically sophisticated, high-risk business which, when running properly, saves lives, makes sick people well, and through the use of diagnostic imaging and therapeutic radiology, discovers and treats pathologies before they become life threatening. However, when the system breaks down, lives can be lost, patient recovery can be compromised, and life-threatening diseases can go undetected.

All imaging centers—whether centers within larger facilities, single rooms in physicians' offices, or freestanding institutions—must be prepared to deal with the ethical and legal considerations related to diagnostic and therapeutic radiology. High-quality patient care, individual autonomy, technical advances, and the established standard of care are but a few of the points that must be recognized by the facility management and staff. Some of these issues can be addressed through the development of policies and procedures for the way the facility is to deliver quality care. All of the facility's employees should be aware of the policies and the importance of compliance. Management must address concerns about policies and procedures, regularly review the policies with all employees, and promptly communicate any changes that will affect the delivery of care or patient safety.

Risk management and safety programs should be designed and implemented to decrease liability, minimize risk, and protect the facility's good name. While these programs may appear on the surface to be self-serving, when they are applied to the practices of the center, the quality of patient care will increase and the risk to patient and employee safety will decrease. A safe and productive environment is the objective of every health care provider; therefore, the implementation of risk management and safety programs will assist the facility in reaching one of its key goals.

Administration in the health care setting must draft employment policies that will protect the facility and the employee. Personnel must be informed of job and professional expectations at the time of employment, and management must be prepared to enforce policies in a fair and equitable manner across all levels of the workforce.

Everyone involved in health care must understand the rights of the consumer patient. Delivery of services should center around the patient's well-being, as well as the accepted and expected standard of care. Educated consumers force health care providers into the roles of educators and gatekeepers. To meet the demands of these professional roles, all personnel should be aware of policies and procedures that affect the delivery of care, new technological advances that enable more accurate diagnosis and treatment, and the ever-changing needs of the population and the profession. Understanding these responsibilities will create a stronger provider–consumer patient relationship and subsequently a more efficient and effective health care delivery system.

# Ethics in Imaging and Therapy

Ann M. Obergfell

**H**ealth care has become a complex system of sophisticated diagnostic tests followed by tried, effective or experimental treatments, which may cure the patient, relieve pain, or prolong life. The system requires that providers and consumer patients make many decisions concerning the course and process of treatment. Decisions concerning when to treat, how to treat, how long to treat, and who will make the decisions concerning treatment are just a few of the issues that must be resolved.

Ethical considerations play a role in all aspects of health care delivery. Some issues, such as who will make decisions and how care will be delivered, appear to have black-and-white answers. However, these and many other health care questions are not easy and may not have "right" answers. Health care providers are bombarded by such questions, the equivocating response to which may be a complicated mixture of judgments based on social morals, religious values, and public policy.

Review of ethical principles and professional codes of ethics will help radiologic science professionals understand their responsibility to the patient, the general public, and the profession.

## ETHICS DEFINED

Many authors have attempted to define ethics through the use of religious theory and moral practice. Others define ethics based on a public policy perception of the difference between right and wrong. A more accurate description falls somewhere in between. Ethics is the study of the standards of conduct and moral judgment, as well as the system or code of morals of a particular group or profession.[1]

Before one can understand the ethical requirements of the radiologic science disciplines, basic ethical theories and principles must be reviewed.

## ETHICAL THEORIES

Two major ethical theories are generally used to analyze ethical dilemmas. These theories view the dilemma from different reference points and, after analysis, may come up with very different results. The first theory, utilitarianism, states that the purpose of all actions should be to bring about the greatest good for the greatest number.[2] The second theory, deontology, is the study of duty or moral obligation based on rules and order.

### Utilitarianism

*Utilitarianism* is an ethical theory that states that the rightness of an action is measured by its consequences.[3] Appropriate outcomes are the most important aspect of the theory, and all actions are measured by the positive or negative results. Cost-benefit analysis is used to judge whether actions are acceptable or will be beneficial to society. If the outcomes of a particular action are positive, the utilitarian will claim that the action benefits society and therefore was a good or acceptable action. If the results are negative, the action is deemed unacceptable and is rejected as inappropriate. A utilitarian may deem it acceptable to lie to a patient, for example, if the result of that action is beneficial and the patient is not harmed.

One problem with a consequence-driven ethical theory is that the individual's value or personal importance may cloud interpretation of whether the outcomes are positive or negative. Unless each individual's worth is valued equally, those who society may deem to be of lesser value—such as the poor, the mentally ill, and the disabled—may lose out when placed in competition with more "valued" members of society.[4] For example, if an action is designed to benefit the disabled and if nondisabled members of society must pay a price for the action, the action may be viewed as having a negative result and therefore deemed unacceptable.

### Deontology

The second ethical theory, known as *deontology,* or the *deontological theory,* reviews a situation based on the relevant rules. Consequences are generally not taken into consideration or are seen as secondary to the rules guiding the action. An individual who follows this theory would claim that lying to a patient is unacceptable and therefore should never be done even if the patient would benefit from the lie.[5]

Like utilitarianism, deontology may have a negative impact when viewed in light of all the circumstances. Basing a decision on a specific set of rules may prove too rigid and may not allow for conflict between rules. Specific circumstances surrounding a situation also may not fit within the applicable rules, and therefore those rules may not or should not be applied. For example, if the rule is not to kill another, but if a person kills another while defending his or her own life or the life of a loved one, should the absolute rule of not killing be applied to determine ethical value? Likewise, in the area of medical ethics, dilemmas arise over questions such as "Is the withdrawal of life support the same as killing?" or "Is the refusal to initiate a life support system an instance of killing?" Should the absolute rule "Thou shall not kill" apply in these situations? These questions may be answered differently depending on the circumstances surrounding a particular incident. Applying a deontological theory of absolute rules to these questions may result in an inappropriate or unacceptable outcome.

## ETHICAL PRINCIPLES

Several ethical rights and principles come into play in the day-to-day activities of health care delivery. Each principle has a very specific meaning but can be applied to various dilemmas that arise in the health care system.

### Autonomy

Under the principle of *autonomy*, each person is entitled to determine his own destiny with due regard to the individual's considered evaluation and view of the world. Individuals have the basic right of self-determination and should be permitted to make decisions concerning their bodies, in particular, the course of health care diagnosis and treatment.[6]

The radiologic science professional may be placed in the midst of a conflict between a patient's wish to refuse and a physician's orders for a procedure or treatment. It is imperative that the technologist act as an advocate for the patient. Advocacy may require the technologist to act as an intermediary between patient and physician.

### Nonmaleficence

*Nonmaleficence* is founded in the ethical principle "to do no harm."[7] This longstanding principle does not require that the individual perform any action; it merely asks that the person not harm another. Nonmaleficence may present some problems when the patient refuses a treatment or procedure and the therapist or technologist knows that forgoing the recommended health plan may bring the patient harm. Electing to do nothing may cause harm to the patient, but performing the procedure without the patient's consent not only violates the patient's right of self-determination but may cause the patient emotional harm. Again, the technologist is faced with a dilemma to which there is no easy answer.

## Beneficence

Remove and prevent evil and harm, *and* do and promote good, define the principle of *beneficence*.[8] Beneficence differs from nonmaleficence in that it requires the individual to perform some action either to prevent harm or to do good. This may require a health care professional to take a stand against another or to intercede for the patient's well-being.

For example, when a physician's order runs contrary to the patient's wishes, the technologist may have to intercede for the patient by speaking with the physician or by discussing the problem with the appropriate supervisory personnel.

## Justice

The *justice* principle requires that individuals be treated according to what is due, fair, or owed.[9] Some consider this to mean that there be an equal distribution of all benefits. Although equal distribution sounds like a fair principle, it may inadvertently disadvantage a particular group or class. Those individuals who already have less access to health care because of poverty, environment, or locale may suffer if there is an equal distribution, since those who already have care will receive an additional benefit—thus widening the gap between the haves and the have-nots.

Treating individuals by what is due, fair, or owed again requires the decision maker to set aside preconceived ideas concerning personal worth. Failing to set aside these ideas may force an individual to make a decision based on what an individual can offer society rather than on what society owes the individual. Therefore, a person who cannot work because of illness or disability may be denied care because he or she is unable to be a contributing member of society. If the justice principle were applied in its purest sense, the disadvantaged and disenfranchised members of society would receive little or no benefit.

## Paternalism

Under the principle of *paternalism*, a person treats another in the same way that a parent treats a child.[10] Health care has a long history of following this principle. Since the beginning, physicians have diagnosed patients' illnesses and identified the plan for treatment. The patient had no role in the decision-making process and often was not given information concerning the course of diagnosis and treatment. Although this practice is slowly changing with the advent of recognized patient rights,[11] in many cases, health care providers still play a paternalistic role when dealing with patients.

In diagnostic imaging, patients enter a facility with little, if any, knowledge of why they have been sent there or what they should expect. Their concerns may be overlooked or disregarded because the health care provider "knows what is best" for the patient and becomes more concerned with completing the procedure or treatment than dealing with the patient's apprehensions.

## Fidelity

The principle of *fidelity* requires that the professional be faithful to the patient's reasonable expectations. The patient expects the professional to (1) meet the basic needs of the patient, including the need for privacy and modesty; (2) be a competent professional; (3) follow the policies and procedures of the facility; (4) abide by agreements made with the patient, such as consent and refusal; and (5) abide by the code of ethics developed by the professional organization.[12]

The reasonable expectations of a patient can generally be met if the professional understands the patient's fundamental rights and the profession's code of ethics, which defines appropriate professional behavior.

## PROFESSIONAL ETHICS

Organizations have developed ethical standards or codes of professional responsibility to guide their members in the practice of the discipline. The American Medical Association (AMA) defined a code for its physician members entitled "Principles of Medical Ethics,"[13] and the American Bar Association (ABA) drafted the "Model Code of Professional Responsibility,"[14] which guides attorneys as they practice law. Each of these organizations identified ideals that assist a competent professional making decisions and dealing with patients, clients, and colleagues in the day-to-day practice of the profession.

The American Society of Radiologic Technologists (ASRT) developed a "Code of Ethics for Radiologic Technologists" to guide individuals practicing in the radiologic sciences. The code has several principles which highlight the qualities exemplified by a competent imaging or therapy specialist. Likewise, the Canadian Association of Medical Radiation Technologists (CAMRT), recognizing its obligation to identify and promote professional standards of conduct and performance, established a code of ethics for its members.

## Code of Ethics

The codes of ethics developed by the American Society of Radiologic Technologists and the Canadian Association of Medical Radiation Technologists help guide the professional activities of radiologic science professionals. Recognizing that professional decisions made by radiologic technologists will affect the diagnosis of disease, the selection of future treatment plans, and the rendering of treatment which may cure or relieve pain in the patient, a number of principles to direct the decision-making process were drafted.

Many radiologic science professionals do not understand the importance of their role in health care delivery. Therefore, the principles outlined in the codes of ethics help define and direct the technologist in the daily practice of diagnostic imaging and therapeutic radiology. The codes are designed to encompass all areas of the radiologic sciences and are recognized as the defining principles for all branches of the discipline.

The ASRT and CAMRT codes of ethics both have ten principles which define the personal responsibilities of the radiologic science professional. The following overview of the ASRT Code of Ethics, with the CAMRT companion statement when applicable, will help focus our discussion of ethical responsibilities to the patient, the general public, and the profession.

### Principle One

**The Radiologic Technologist conducts himself/herself in a professional manner, responds to patients' needs and supports colleagues and associates in providing quality patient care.**

*ASRT*

**. . . cooperate with other health care providers . . .**

*CAMRT*

**. . . encourage the trust and confidence of the public through high standards of professional competence, conduct and appearance . . .**

*CAMRT*

The first principle dictates the manner in which the individual conducts himself or herself as a member of the profession. The technologist is expected to respond in an empathetic, yet efficient, way to the patient's needs. Radiologic science professionals must be competent in their delivery of health care services and must encourage colleagues to provide quality care for all patients.

Professional appearance in both dress and demeanor are essential aspects of a competent and caring health professional. Failure to meet these standards by way of an unkempt appearance or unprofessional behavior in the health care setting may signify that the individual does not respect the patient or the profession. The patient's confidence in the caregiver will increase when the technologist maintains a professional attitude throughout the procedure or treatment. The respect of other health care providers can come only after the technologist or therapist has demonstrated through appearance and action that the desired respect is deserved.

## Principle Two

> The Radiologic Technologist acts to advance the principle objective of the profession to provide services to humanity with full respect for the dignity of mankind.
>
> *ASRT*

Radiologic technologists must always respect the dignity of the individual and remember that patients who come to imaging and therapy facilities are at a very vulnerable time in their lives. Each patient should be given absolute and undivided attention. Specific concerns should be addressed immediately and should not be brushed aside or disregarded as unimportant. A patient's modesty and personal dignity must always be respected.

## Principle Three

> The Radiologic Technologist delivers patient care and service unrestricted by the concerns of personal attributes or the nature of the disease or illness, and without discrimination regardless of sex, race, creed, religion, or socioeconomic status.
>
> *ASRT*

> . . . provide service with dignity and respect to all people regardless of race, national or ethnic origin, colour, sex, religion, age, type of illness, mental or physical challenges.
>
> *CAMRT*

As members of the health care team, radiologic technologists must deliver care to all patients, regardless of age, race, gender, religion, nature of illness, or mental or physical disability. This particular principle answers one of the most frequently asked questions in health care: "Do I have to work on the HIV-positive or AIDS patient?" Every member of the profession has an obligation to provide courteous, competent care for each patient who enters the imaging or therapy department. The technologist or therapist must overcome the fear of AIDS and recognize that, through the use of universal precautions, maximum protection from transmission can be achieved. Allowing personal fear to interfere with the ability to provide quality care to the patient is a direct violation of the ethical codes and the patient's individual rights.

## Principle Four

> The Radiologic Technologist practices technology founded upon theoretical knowledge and concepts, utilizes equipment and accessories consistent with the purposes for which they have been designed, and employs procedures and techniques appropriately.
>
> *ASRT*

Members of the radiologic science professions must always practice skills founded on strong scientific theory and utilize equipment for the purposes for which it is designed, through methods prescribed by the manufacturer. Procedures and treatments should follow accepted protocols, because deviations from accepted scientific standards may endanger the well-being of patient, technologist, and other health care professionals.

Radiologic science professionals must understand that they are part of a dynamic, constantly changing health care discipline. Professionals who continue to use techniques that were part of their early professional education, and which have subsequently been rendered obsolete or have been replaced by safer, more efficient, more effective methods, are not meeting the responsibilities of the profession.

## Principle Five

> The Radiologic Technologist assesses situations, exercises care, discretion and judgment, assumes responsibility for professional decisions, and acts in the best interest of the patient.
>
> *ASRT*

The radiologic technologist must take responsibility for all professional decisions. While technologists and therapists work with physicians, each is responsible for his or her own decisions, judgments, and behavior.

Good judgment requires the professional to ask for clarification on orders that do not make sense or do not seem appropriate in light of the patient's condition or history. To follow orders blindly or to perform unwarranted procedures violates the professional's obligation always to act in the patient's best interests.

## Principle Six

> The Radiologic Technologist acts as an agent through observation and communication to obtain pertinent information for the physician to aid in the diagnosis and treatment management of the patient, and recognizes that interpretation and diagnosis are outside the scope of practice for the profession.
>
> *ASRT*

> . . . be mindful that patients must seek diagnostic information from their treating physician. In those instances where a discreet comment to the appropriate authority may assist diagnosis or treatment, the technologist may feel morally obliged to provide one.
>
> *CAMRT*

Radiologic technologists must obtain information from all patients who undergo tests or treatments in an imaging or therapy department. It is not enough merely to ask questions of patients or their representatives; the patient's mannerisms and movements must also be observed and noted to accurately assess the patient.

The information received through questioning and observation can first be utilized to determine how the technologist will perform the procedure through adaptations of position, equipment, and technical factors. A technologist must understand how to adjust standard technique based on body habitus and pathologic processes.[15] For example, to acquire a quality radiograph on a patient with a history of emphysema, the technologist will utilize different exposure factors than on a patient who enters with a pleural effusion. Without asking history and assessing the patient, it would be impossible to adjust technical factors and obtain optimum radiographs. Relying on automatic exposure controls and phototimers for technical variations violates the patient's right to competent and professional care.

The information obtained from the patient should be given to the radiologist or other physician before the interpretation or diagnostic stage of the procedure. A radiologist should not perform any fluoroscopic study until information concerning the patient's age, history, condition, and current complaints have been reported and discussed. A diagnosis should not be made until the physician has the patient's history. In the case of a trauma patient, any information concerning the incident, such as whether it was a head-on collision or a fall from a particular height, will assist the physician during interpretation and diagnosis.[16] If the physician responsible for interpretation does not have adequate history concerning the patient, he or she may overlook or fail to recognize pathology.

Although it is beyond the scope of practice for technologists and therapists to interpret and diagnose, it is imperative that they, as the gatekeepers of information concerning the patient, understand and follow the ethical requirements of observation, assessment, and evaluation.

## *Principle Seven*

> **The Radiologic Technologist utilizes equipment and accessories, employs techniques and procedures, performs services in accordance with an accepted standard of practice, and demonstrates expertise in limiting the radiation exposure to the patient, self, and other members of the health care team.**
>
> *ASRT*

> **Conduct all technical procedures with due regard to current radiation safety standards.**
>
> *CAMRT*

The radiologic technologist must understand and provide services to the patient based on the current accepted standard of care for the profession. Radiographic equipment is housed in a variety of settings, ranging from sophisticated, high-tech medical centers to small rural offices. Regardless of the location of the equipment, it is the technologist's responsibility to utilize the available equipment according to the accepted standards and regulations. Examples of accepted standards include but are not limited to the utilization of compatible film screen combinations to obtain the best images with the least amount of radiation exposure[17]; development and adoption of accurate technique charts for each piece of equipment on site[18]; availability and use of appropriate shielding devices and collimation to the correct field size on all patients; cleaning of the equipment, including screens and cassettes, on a regular basis[19]; performance of repeat analysis studies on a continuing basis, with a mechanism for taking corrective measures when a problem is identified[20]; and consistent monitoring and maintenance of the film processor.[21]

Compliance with current radiation safety standards is one of the most important components of practice in the diagnostic imaging and therapeutic sciences. Professionals in these fields are deemed experts in the application of radiation for diagnostic and therapeutic purposes. With expert status comes the underlying responsibility to protect the patient and the general public from unnecessary exposure to radiation.

Deviation from the appropriate radiation safety or technical standards not only violates the codes of ethics but denies the patient the safe and high-quality health care services that are expected and deserved.

## Principle Eight

> **The Radiologic Technologist practices ethical conduct appropriate to the profession and protects the patient's right to quality radiologic technology care.**
>
> *ASRT*

To meet this ethical principle, a radiologic science professional should maintain a good, positive attitude about the profession by understanding the importance of the role of the technologist or therapist in the delivery of quality patient care; practice professional communication not only with the patient but also with other members of the health care team; develop strong interpersonal skills to be used when dealing with patients, peers, and members of the general public; and respect the dignity of the individual regardless of condition or social status.

Radiologic science professionals have an obligation to respect the patient's rights and to protect the unknowing patient from unethical, inappropriate, or illegal practices. Violation of this responsibility may occur when the technologist or therapist fails to ask, receive, and document an appropriate history, including pregnancy when applicable, from every patient who enters the facility. Performing the wrong procedure, charging for films, supplies, or procedures that have not been used or ordered, or inappropriately sharing confidential information not only violate ethical principles but may cross the line into illegal activity for which the technologist may be personally liable.

## Principle Nine

> **The Radiologic Technologist respects confidences entrusted in the course of professional practice, respects the patient's right to privacy, and reveals confidential information only as required by law or to protect the welfare of the individual or the community.**
>
> *ASRT*

> **Preserve and protect the confidentiality of any information, either medical or personal, acquired through professional contact with the patient. An exception may be appropriate when the disclosure of such information is necessary to the treatment of the patient,**

the safety of other patients or health care providers,
or is a legal requirement.

*CAMRT*

Radiologic science professionals are obligated to protect the patient's
privacy and to keep information confidential unless the law or the patient's well-being requires disclosure. Legal disclosure is generally limited
to cases of suspected abuse and reporting of communicable diseases if
required under state statute. If statutory disclosure is required in the jurisdiction, the health care provider who reports according to the guidelines
is generally protected from liability. Reporting mechanisms must be followed in the manner proscribed by law. Health care facilities should develop policies and procedures that address these laws and must educate
all employees who may be involved in the reporting process. Disclosure
that does not meet the requirements of the law may subject the reporting
individual to liability for breach of patient confidentiality.

A technologist may also be required to disclose information concerning
a patient's statements if the patient claims that he or she intends to harm
a specific individual and appears capable of following through with the
threat.[22] A general threat or complaint made by an unhappy patient is
not the same as a specific threat regarding an identifiable individual and
therefore need not be reported to the authorities.

Radiologic science professionals must be alert to and aware of anything
that the patient says or does. Ignoring the patient or not concentrating on
the individual may cause the technologist to miss some important piece of
information which may protect either the patient, as in the case of suspected abuse, or the general public, in the case of a patient who makes
a threat and is able to follow through. The ability to use good judgment
will assist the technologist in meeting the requirements of this ethical
principle.

## Principle Ten

The Radiologic Technologist continually strives to improve knowledge and skill by participating in educational and professional activities, sharing knowledge
with colleagues and investigating new and innovative
aspects of professional practice. One means available
to improve knowledge and skill is through professional continuing education.

*ASRT*

Advance the art and science of medical radiation technology through ongoing professional development . . .

*CAMRT*

**Recognize the participation and support of our association is a professional responsibility.**

*CAMRT*

The radiologic sciences are constantly changing, and technological advances are made every day. A responsible technologist maintains competency in the profession by staying current. The most effective method for remaining current in the discipline is to attend and actively participate in professional educational conferences, to read professional journals and trade publications, and to provide and share information on the discipline with colleagues both in and out of the profession. Within facilities, an active and consistent in-service program prepared by members of the department will allow for the sharing of information. Presentations on the newest technological innovations, professional achievements, and current health care delivery concerns, as well as facility policy and procedures, can all be incorporated into a quality in-service program.

Participation in professional organizations is not only of great importance; it is an ethical obligation for technologists and therapists. These organizations are responsible for coordinating, changing, and protecting the interests of the radiologic sciences. Activities ranging from coordinating and lobbying for licensing or certification laws, protecting the unsuspecting public from excessive or inappropriate radiation exposure, preparing and developing curricula for educational programs, encouraging research activities, and providing continuing education for their memberships are but a few of the myriad responsibilities of a strong professional organization.

The strength of the organization will come from its members. Active participation by all radiologic science professionals will lend credibility to the activities of the profession and will help create an environment to advance the concerns of all. Professionals differ from common laborers in that they are bound together by common interests, education, and experience. Choosing to become a professional requires a commitment not only to the day-to-day activities of the job, but a life-long commitment to education, intellectual growth, and the advancement of the discipline. The best way to meet these requirements is to belong to and actively participate in the activities of professional organizations at the state, province, or national level.

## OTHER IMPORTANT ETHICAL CONSIDERATIONS

**Practice only those procedures for which the necessary qualifications are held unless such procedures have been properly delegated by an appropriate medi-**

cal authority and for which the technologist has received adequate training to an acceptable level of competence.

*CAMRT*

. . . practice only those disciplines of medical radiation technology for which he or she has been certified by the CAMRT and is currently competent.

*CAMRT*

The complex nature of the radiologic science disciplines requires that individuals generally practice in one or two areas of specialization. True competency in all areas would be virtually impossible for even the most outstanding technologist or therapist. A technologist who, for whatever reason, elects to practice in an area for which he or she has not met the educational or certification requirements may confront ethical and legal violations he or she is unprepared to answer.

Cross-training in the radiologic sciences demands more than teaching someone which button to push or which knob to turn. The extensive educational requirements of patient care, physics, equipment, anatomy, physiology, and pathology are evidenced by the type of questions asked on the advanced certification examinations. It would not be appropriate for a family practice physician to perform neurosurgery if he had not met the appropriate educational requirements; likewise, a radiographer should not attempt to perform cardiovascular interventional or nuclear medicine studies without the requisite skill and education. The general public expects and deserves more from those to whom they entrust their care.

## CONCLUSION

Ethical questions abound in the radiologic sciences, and it is clear that there are no easy answers to many of them. Through codes of ethics the profession has given a framework to direct, coordinate, and assist the technologist practicing in the challenging and constantly changing health care delivery system. Radiologic science professionals must understand codes of ethics, abide by their principles, and respect the individual autonomy and dignity of the patient.

## N O T E S

1. *Webster's New World Dictionary of the American Language,* 2nd ed. (New York: Simon and Schuster, 1982).
2. Ibid.

3. Tom L. Beauchamp and James E. Childress, *Principles of Biomedical Ethics*, 4th ed. (New York: Oxford University Press, 1994).
4. Ruth Purtillo, *Ethical Dimensions in the Health Professions* (Philadelphia: Saunders, 1993).
5. Purtillo, *Ethical Dimensions*, 10.
6. Robert A. Buerke and Louis D. Vottero, "Ethical and Legal Issues," in *Introduction to Radiography and Patient Care*, ed. Adler and Carlton (Philadelphia: Saunders, 1994).
7. Purtillo, *Ethical Dimensions*, 19.
8. *Webster's*.
9. Beauchamp and Childress.
10. Ibid.
11. American Hospital Association, *A Patient's Bill of Rights*, adopted 1973, revised 1992.
12. Purtillo, *Ethical Dimensions*, 42.
13. American Medical Association, "Principles of Medical Ethics," in Beauchamp and Childress (Chapter 1).
14. American Bar Association, "Model Code of Professional Responsibility" (National Center for Professional Responsibility and the American Bar Association, 1981), in *Selected Statutes, Rules, & Standards on the Legal Profession* (St. Paul, MN: West Publishing Co., 1987).
15. Stewart C. Bushong, *Radiologic Science for Technologists: Physics, Biology, and Protection*, 5th ed. (St. Louis: Mosby-Yearbook, 1993), 304–320.
16. Michael W. Drafke, *Trauma and Mobile Radiography* (Philadelphia: Davis, 1990).
17. Bushong, *Radiologic Science*.
18. Ibid.
19. Ibid., Chapter 13, 231.
20. Joel Gray et al., *Quality Control in Diagnostic Imaging* (Baltimore: University Park Press, 1983), 27–32.
21. Raymond P. Rossi, "Performance Evaluation of Film Processors in the Clinical Environment," in *Film Processing in Medical Imaging*, ed. Arthur G. Haus (Madison, WI: Medical Physics Publishing, 1993), 103–114.
22. Tarasoff v. Regents of the University of California, 551 P.2d 334 (1976).

# 3

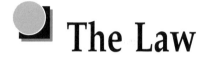

# The Law

Angeline Golden

The purpose of this chapter is to provide a brief overview of the structure that regulates, controls, restricts, punishes, and compensates individual behavior and interaction among individuals within a society. It is that
intangible social structure that has developed over time, through trial and
error, and reflects each society's particular values. This structure is commonly referred to as the *legal system* or the *law*.

It is also the purpose of this chapter to show—through examples from
actual cases or from state laws—how this society's legal system affects the
*medical practitioner*—specifically, the practitioner in the field of diagnostic
imaging and therapeutic radiology.[1]

## THE EVOLUTION OF ORDER

Conflict is inevitable wherever groups of people live together or come
in contact with one another on a regular or sporadic basis. History has
demonstrated that such groups, both large and small, create or adopt external systems of control to regulate human behavior in order to minimize
conflict. For example, some political groupings known as states write documents commonly referred to as constitutions, which form governments
to conduct the business of a nation:

> **We the People of the United States, in Order to form a
> more perfect Union, establish Justice, insure domestic
> Tranquility, provide for the common defence, promote the
> general Welfare, and secure the Blessings of Liberty to
> ourselves and our posterity, do ordain and establish this
> Constitution for the United States of America.[2]**

Colleges or universities write charters to conduct the business of education and to regulate student behavior during matriculation; religious institutions develop written articles of faith to govern their members; and hospitals formulate articles of incorporation and adopt by-laws to conduct their affairs.

The end products of these formal systems developed to control or regulate the behavior of group members are called *laws, rules,* or *codes.* These laws define conduct that is acceptable or prohibited. They may also establish a predetermined method of resolving conflict and may set forth punishments for unacceptable conduct. For example, a state may choose to regulate the practice of medicine by requiring a physician to obtain a license to practice.[3] If a physician practices without obtaining the required document, he or she may face sanctions from the state but may also be able to take advantage of a predetermined procedure for resolving the dispute.[4]

**Laws, like houses, lean on one another.**

*Edmund Burke (1729–1797)*
*Irish philosopher, statesman*

As was previously stated, but is worth reemphasizing, *laws develop over time.* In the United States, our legal system includes laws brought from England by the early English colonists (the *common law*).[5] These laws had in turn developed over time in England by the influence of invading armies, by competing interests between the people, by the Crown, by the church, and by the gradual evolution of judicial wisdom.

In this country, laws pertaining to whether or not a physician or other health professional can be charged with medical malpractice have also evolved slowly. These laws have culminated in certain requirements, such as that a lawsuit must be brought against a physician within a specific period of time (commonly known as a *statute of limitations*[6]), but only after a reasonable inquiry has been made prior to bringing the lawsuit.[7]

The term *malpractice* encompasses the legal concept of *negligence.* Before a determination can be made of whether a physician is negligent in her delivery of care in a particular circumstance, the applicable standard of care must be examined. The standard of care for a physician may vary from state to state or from jurisdiction to jurisdiction, but in general, it refers to the level of care given by a physician in the same or similar circumstances. The physician "must have and use the knowledge, skill, and care ordinarily possessed and employed by members of the profession in good standing."[8]

If we examine the duty of a radiologist when dealing with a patient, it is easy to see how laws addressing that duty have evolved over time. When x-rays were first used to diagnose and treat illness, it was unknown what harm could result from incorrect procedures. Now it is known that x-rays can harm a fetus. A physician who fails to determine in a routine situation whether a female patient is pregnant before ordering her to be x-rayed may be found to have violated the accepted standard of care and therefore held liable (financially accountable) for any harm suffered by the pregnant patient or by her offspring as a result of the radiation exposure.[9]

## DEFINITIONS OF LAW

There are numerous definitions of the term *law*. Some are amusing:

> **The law is sort of hocus pocus science, that smiles in yer face while it picks your pocket.**
>
> *Charles Macklin (1697–1797)*
> *Irish actor, dramatist*

> **If the law supposes that, said Mr. Bumble, "the law is a ass, a idiot."**
>
> *Charles Dickens*, Oliver Twist

Some are ponderous:

> **The law in its majestic equality, forbids rich and poor alike to sleep under bridges, beg in the streets, or steal bread.**
>
> *Anatole France (1844–1924)*

And some are moralistic:

> **The good of the people is the greatest law.**
>
> *Cicero (106–43 B.C.)*

Law in its generic sense is defined as a "body of rules of action or conduct prescribed by controlling authority, and having binding legal force," represented as the "solemn expression of will of the supreme power of the State" and "that which must be obeyed and followed by citizens subject to sanctions or legal consequences."[10]

While the concept of the law is an intangible, there are tangibles that have resulted directly from people's attempts to activate that concept. For example, informed consent documents must be explained to a patient and signed by the patient or a personal representative of the patient before certain diagnostic tests or therapeutic procedures may be conducted (see Appendixes). Other examples of tangibles include voice-activated dictating machines, which were invented and developed in part for the use of physicians dictating medical reports and for lawyers to accurately transcribe a witness's testimony during a deposition (oral interrogation or questioning). Physical structures such as jury rooms, where a jury retires to deliberate the facts of a case in order to arrive at a verdict, are other examples of such tangibles.

It is not an overstatement to say that virtually *every* aspect of the medical practitioner's educational and professional life will be affected by both the intangible concept of the law and the tangible manifestations of that idea. The interweaving of law and medicine in American society requires the medical professional—whether radiologist or radiographer, medical school professor or vocational teacher, designer or manufacturer of x-ray equipment, hospital administrator or supervisor of radiographers—to have an understanding of how the legal system *mandates certain standards of care in the performance of professional duties.*

The very fact that most readers of this text either are now, or soon will be, licensed medical practitioners in a professional specialty, indicates exposure to certain laws or regulations that control practice. The schools in which professionals are educated, the hospitals in which they practice, and the physicians who order procedures are regulated by either state laws, local ordinances, or administrative regulations which dictate specific requirements as to funding, size of student or patient population, hospital location, training, licensing, insurability, and many other aspects of education and health care delivery.

Upon completion of an educational program, the legal system continues to regulate both individual and group behavior through medical licensing or certification. Health professionals are required in many states to complete continuing education credits on a regular basis.[11] Professionals registered by the American Registry of Radiologic Technologists (ARRT) must meet certain continuing education requirements to remain on the registry. Hospitals and schools must undergo periodic evaluations from regulators and accrediting agencies.

Medical professional behavior is further regulated when lawsuits are filed as a result of the negligent performance of duties. Ask *any* medical professional who has been sued what impact that lawsuit has had on his or her professional behavior.

The foregoing is admittedly only a cursory view. A multitude of books, articles, and published judicial decisions are available in law, medical, and public libraries for more in-depth exploration of the subject.

The following is a brief synopsis—by lighthearted example—of how the major broad categories of the law develop.

## CRIMINAL AND CIVIL LAW

**Criminal Law:**   The substantive criminal law is that law which, for the purpose of preventing harm to society, (a) declares what conduct is criminal and (b) prescribes the punishment to be imposed for such conduct.[12]

**Civil Law:**    Laws concerned with civil or private rights and remedies.[13]

Ideally, a democratic society will decide through its various representatives the rules to control its individual members. As an example, consider rock and roll music, arising in our American musical heritage in the last half of this century. There is no question that society in general has accepted such music. But assume that a certain community has deplored the loudness of rock and roll and passed laws regulating such music which is so noisy or vibratory that it is considered harmful to others.

Imagine that a band playing next door at 3:00 A.M. disturbs a person's sleep. The individual who is affected by the music is aware that the community has passed laws prohibiting loud music in a residential area between 12:00 A.M. and 7:00 A.M. (or at any time the noise is so loud that it disturbs the peace). Feeling disoriented and exhausted, the individual registers a complaint with local law enforcement officials. If upon investigation the police find that the music is too loud, a charge will be filed in the criminal courts alleging a violation of the law banning the playing of loud music after hours.

Assume that the law which has been violated has been classified by the state as a criminal law. A criminal law is meant for the protection of *all* society within a geographic community, not just for the protection of a single individual. Therefore, although one individual was affected by the loud music, he becomes a victim or a witness to the fact that society as a whole has been wronged. The noise makers must therefore be punished by the state that has made the law (*State v. Noise Makers* or *People versus Loud Band*).

Within the same example, let's assume that the music was so loud that it damaged the person's eardrum, and he therefore decides to consult with his lawyer. The lawyer informs her client that he has personally suffered a civil wrong; that is, apart from the noise makers' criminal act, some "duty" may exist on their part not to cause injury to others. The lawyer explains that, where such a duty exists, it was breached when the eardrum ruptured. The cost for the repair of the eardrum is a part of the "damage" suffered. And, if it can be shown that the ruptured eardrum was in fact caused by the noise makers, this cost should be rightfully borne by them—even if their intent at 3:00 A.M. was only to entertain house guests and not to rupture their neighbor's eardrum. In contrast to criminal law, civil law now applies because the individual alone will be compensated *for the injury*, not all of society. The injured person becomes the plaintiff or the complainant, and the noise makers have become the defendants in a civil lawsuit (*Mr. A. Hurt Eardrum, Plaintiff v. Evil Noise Makers, Defendants*).

## CONSTITUTIONAL LAW

**Constitutional Law:** "That branch of the public law of a nation or state which treats of the organization, powers and frame of government. . . ."[14]

The compact, agreement, or master plan considered by a society when establishing itself as a formal body is usually called a *constitution*. It may be likened to the largest common denominator, inclusive of all individually enumerated rights, which seeks not to abridge any of those rights unless done so within stated parameters. For example, the Constitution of the United States protects individual expressions of speech, assembly, and religion unless for some reason the higher good of the country or state permits them to be abridged for specific reasons. (One cannot stand and freely scream, "Fire!" in a crowded theater.)

Within the framework of its constitution, a society's representatives— the legislature—constantly enact or repeal laws so as to further the society's governmental interests (again, while attempting to preserve the constitutionally given rights of individuals). Continuing with our imaginary rock music example, that society's constitution may permit people to have the right to assemble at any time. So the loud noise makers may argue, "We assembled, played good music for those who wanted to listen— and the constitution says we can. Therefore, the local law, restricting our playing after 11:00 P.M., is unconstitutional because it violates our right to assemble, as well as our right of free speech." The noise makers then bring their own lawsuit on constitutional grounds, alleging that their constitutional right has been violated.

## ADMINISTRATIVE LAW

**Administrative Law:** Body of law created by administrative agencies in the form of rules, regulations, orders, and decisions.[15]

The legislature, or congress, decides that, rather than dictating when loud music may or may not be played, it should pass a bill stating that *all* loud music is unlawful, but leaves it to the "secretary of music and noise" to define loud music. This passing of power to decide matters from a statutory body to an agency or department is known as *delegation*. The legislature presumes that the secretary is knowledgeable in the area of music and will draft regulations that are both acceptable and reasonable. Laws and regulations so drafted are within the realm of administrative law.

Although all of the above is simplistic and based on a rather far-fetched example, the purpose is to demonstrate a few basic concepts of the very broad discipline known as the law.

Health care regulation has also evolved over time to control the activity of health care practitioners. Let us now consider the practice of radiologic technology. A radiographer at a large metropolitan hospital interacts all day with doctors, hospital administrators, nurses, and other technologists. The radiographer takes orders, gives orders, observes and interacts with patients, and records professional actions. Who makes the rules concerning these activities? From the moment an employee arrives in the hospital's parking lot, rules guide behavior. Who decides where people will park? Who decides when it's time to go home? Who decides when conduct is less than professional? Is it professional to spit on the floor? Who says not to? Does it even need to be said? When differences arise, how are they to be resolved?

For example, if a state law prohibits the administration of pharmaceuticals by anyone other than a physician or registered nurse and a radiographer administers medication, even on the order of a physician, he or she may be liable for any injury to the patient resulting from that action. If the prohibitive statute carries a criminal penalty and the radiographer is found guilty of violating the statute, the radiographer may be required to pay a fine or be incarcerated for a period of time dictated by the statute. The radiographer may also be held civilly liable and may be required to financially compensate the injured patient. If an administrative agency has been given the power to control the practice of radiation machine operators within the state, the agency may determine that this radiographer is unfit to practice professionally and can remove the license or certificate that permits him or her to work within the jurisdiction.

## THE ANATOMY OF A LAWSUIT

In primitive society, direct, physical, confrontational acts resolved problems. However, civilized society has developed laws providing for the nonviolent settlement of differences. In earlier times, truth sometimes hinged on the successful performance of physical acts to ascertain who was telling the truth. These physical acts were known as *trials*. The modern usage of the term *trial* is accorded much the same status; that is, the party who manages to convince a judge or jury of her version of the truth will usually prevail.

One who believes he or she has been wronged and has a "cause of action" against a wrongdoer must still run a gamut of hurdles—the historical term being *feats*. These contemporary hurdles are dictated by specific procedures. The first is to determine exactly the nature of the complaint. For instance, in our example of the ruptured eardrum, the injured person's attorney must investigate the facts to determine whether the law imposes any duty on the band not to rupture the eardrums of unwilling listeners and then whether the ruptured eardrum was actually the result of the loud music played by the alleged lawbreakers. All this must be investigated and accomplished *prior* to the filing of a lawsuit. One must name the correct parties and allege, at least minimally, the facts known at the time of filing. This can be accomplished only after an inquiry. A "reasonable" inquiry into the matter, which demonstrates a legal foundation for bringing the lawsuit, is sufficient and all that is required for a lawsuit in most jurisdictions.[16] Once a reasonable inquiry has been made, a lawsuit may be filed in good faith. The requirement of reasonable inquiry may explain why some in the medical profession have been interviewed, had their hospital records examined, or otherwise been questioned about an event by an attorney, a paralegal, or an insurance adjustor prior to the filing of a lawsuit.

The second hurdle is the lawsuit itself. Who or what individuals should be named as defendants? Which court will have jurisdiction of the case? What matters are to be alleged as the negligent acts causing injuries? What damages have been caused? Were the injuries caused totally by the wrongful conduct? (For example, is it relevant that, because of inadequate radiographs, a doctor failed to diagnose a condition that later resulted in injury or death of a patient? Must the radiographer be named as a defendant in the lawsuit? The radiographer's supervisor? The hospital administrator? The hospital itself? Is there in fact a negligent act to which the death can be traced?

## The Complaint

When considering a lawsuit, it is always important to review it from within the four corners of the originating document, the *complaint*. The complaint will display in an abbreviated fashion the "who, what, where, why, and sometimes how" of the action. The cursory nature of the complaint may leave the defendant with many questions concerning his involvement in the cause of action. Therefore, the plaintiff must develop proof to solidify issues from the sketchy material of the complaint—that is, how he will prove the charges in his complaint.

Some allegations asserted in a complaint are "boilerplate" (standard form) assertions, which are remnants of a past era that encouraged the art of rhetorical, legalized writing over plain language in a legal document.

But over time most jurisdictions have adopted rules of civil procedure that simplify the preparation and language of a complaint. These rules, generally referred to as the "civil rules," instruct attorneys as to the highly rigid and formalistic means of initiating a lawsuit and the precise procedural steps necessary for the conduct of a lawsuit through trial and the appellate process.

Attorneys are not hampered in their preparation of a complaint by matters relating to copyrights or plagiarism. Copying successful complaints is usually encouraged. In fact, most attorneys use form books containing standard complaints when drafting legal documents. Lawyers proudly exchange copies of their complaints with their colleagues. What has developed, much to the chagrin of the nonlawyer world, are documents whose phrases and terms more closely emulate words and statements used by courts or statutory sources than language familiar to the layperson. (See appendixes for sample complaints: form complaints and one specifically drafted for a lawsuit.)

When the defendant receives the complaint, an investigation must begin so that an appropriate answer and defense can be developed. This investigation is the third step of the lawsuit and is generally called the *discovery* period.

## Discovery

Remember, the first step in the lawsuit is the prospective plaintiff's duty to make a reasonable and independent inquiry *prior* to filing the complaint, to ascertain whether an action can properly be brought and maintained against the alleged defendant. Next is the preparation of a complaint that lodges the matter in the appropriate court, with the proper parties identified, and alleges at least a disputable cause of action. (The defendant, upon receipt of a lawsuit filed against him or her must answer within a certain number of days—usually 20—or a default judgment can be obtained against him or her.)

Discovery permits the parties to flesh out the more common elements of what actually occurred before going on to the next stage, the trial.[17] Discovery presents an opportunity to uncover facts, take sworn testimony from parties and witnesses, obtain documentary evidence, ask written questions, get the opinion of experts, and determine whether to attempt to settle or to try the case.

The media world may give high marks to presentations based on the element of surprise; as a moviegoing public, we like courtroom drama. We prefer complex plots with last-minute testimony by surprise witnesses. In the real world, especially in the law, surprise is abhorred.

The first lesson for attorneys in discovery is very simple: no surprises. A failure to be open, a failure to investigate, a failure to avail oneself of the tools of discovery can lead to sanctions, monetary punishments, or loss of a case.

One can analogize an attorney's use of discovery to an actor's approaching opening night. To be believable, the actor must learn as much about the plot as possible; know the props, the stage settings, the lighting, the characters, and the lines—until the time of the performance. A trial is much the same. By the time of the trial, the case should be so thoroughly investigated and analyzed that virtually nothing is left to chance. The selection of a jury and its final composition is the one area in which chance is the most difficult to control. However, if discovery is used to the fullest, jury results can be more predictable. Jury selection is a course in and of itself, and whole texts are available on the subject. It is interesting to know that, in important cases, mock trials are conducted using paid volunteers to "listen" to the case, render a verdict, and answer questions about the presentation. The end result may not be far distant from what a true jury may decide, assuming that discovery has permitted a thorough "dress rehearsal" and the attorney has properly prepared for the matter.[18]

## The Professional as a Party

The question of greatest concern to health professionals is what happens if they are sued or called as witnesses. If a lawsuit has been filed, the professional will receive a summons and a copy of a complaint, which names the party—in this case, the defendant whom the plaintiff has sued. (Remember that, although this chapter references the law of Kentucky, the procedure is generally the same in other states.) The defendant is advised that the law permits twenty days in which to answer the complaint and of the possible penalties for failing to file an answer. The named party should immediately contact an attorney to represent and protect the defendant's interests. Whether working for a hospital, a clinic, or a private physician, the radiographer should be aware of what provisions have been made if an employee is personally sued as a result of professional activities while working for the employer. Many employers will provide legal representation, but some will not. There are a multitude of factors involved in medical negligence or malpractice actions, which are discussed in other chapters of this book. Of necessity, such actions can be discussed only in a cursory fashion in an introductory text, but the health professional should at least be familiar with the legal ramifications of a lawsuit. The health professional should *never* treat a lawsuit lightly. He or she should notify superiors at once and seek the advice of an attorney even if the employer provides representation.

Once representation has been verified, the attorney will guide and direct the defendant's participation in the legal action through its conclusion. He or she will confer with the client, answer questions, and give advice on the proper course based on the best interests of the defendant. This is what the attorney has been trained and paid to do. If the defendant radiographer is sued along with the doctor who ordered the medical procedure, the hospital where the procedure was conducted, and/or the manufacturer of the equipment used, it is imperative to consider obtaining separate counsel. Otherwise, the technologist may become the scapegoat to whom the other defendants point as the responsible party.

Radiographers and other radiologic science professionals should decide if obtaining personal liability insurance is in their best interests. The need for coverage can best be determined by asking what coverage the employer has for the employee and how that coverage will affect the technologist if named separately in a lawsuit. Hospitals, clinics, and offices all maintain different types of coverage for employees. Therefore, it is in the employee's best interests to ascertain the terms of coverage and make an independent judgment about the need for individual coverage.

### The Professional as a Witness

Suppose the radiologic science professional has received a notice to take a deposition "upon oral examination" at a stated time and place. The professional may be considered a witness to an event that is of concern in a filed lawsuit. Perhaps the complaining party, the plaintiff, wants to know if the physician ordered a certain radiographic procedure and wants to determine what the radiographer knows about the procedure. Under the rules of civil procedure, a party may obtain discovery (in this example, by asking questions in person) regarding any matter, not privileged, that is relevant to the subject matter involved in the pending action.[19] The most widely known privilege is the *attorney-client privilege,* which protects communications between attorney and client. Even though the radiographer has not been sued and is merely being asked questions about an event, the witness should have an attorney present to protect his or her best interests. Discussions with the attorney will fall within the "privileged" classification.[20]

It is important to understand that the rules of discovery vary from jurisdiction to jurisdiction and may vary from state courts to federal courts. Thus, specific questions about the local rules of the jurisdiction in which the lawsuit has been filed should be directed to an attorney familiar with the area or may be obtained from a law library or the clerk of the court in the city or county.

## The Deposition

The process of deposition can be very intimidating. Nevertheless, the witness must be prepared to answer all questions in a clear and concise manner. The following synopsis will explain the usual process for deposition of a witness:

**1.** The supervisor or other representative in the facility will inform the radiologic science professional that Dr. Kildare has been sued and that the technologist may be called as a witness to answer questions concerning the procedure requested by the physician. The technologist will probably be asked to review notes and recollections of the incident and discuss this information with a representative of the hospital, perhaps even the hospital's attorney. The technologist will probably also be asked to provide specific details about the event.

**2.**   The technologist will receive a notice or summons to take a deposition "upon oral examination." These documents may be sent by registered or certified mail or delivered by a person such as a special bailiff, process server, or deputy sheriff. This document will explain what the matter concerns, as well as what might happen if the technologist fails to appear at the time and date specified. For example, if a summons has been issued in the Commonwealth of Kentucky to appear for a deposition and if the individual served fails to appear, the person may be held in contempt of court, which could result in a fine or jail time. The document may be entitled a *subpoena duces tecum,* which means that it is asking the witness to bring to the deposition hospital books, records, or personal papers which may have a bearing on the event in question. (See Appendixes for sample forms.)

**3.**   Despite a common misconception, attorneys have learned, either through training or from experience, to be accommodating. The witness will probably have been contacted in advance to determine whether a certain date and time for deposition is acceptable; or if, having received notice without advance arrangement, the witness is unable to attend, he or she will probably be permitted to reschedule where possible. The problem with scheduling depositions is that several persons' schedules must be accommodated—those of all parties to the action, their respective attorneys, and the court reporter or videotape technician who will record the sworn testimony.

**4.**   The technologist must arrive at the deposition as scheduled. Several people will be present: the court reporter, who will make a complete transcript of the event including identifying and swearing of the witness, other parties and their counsel, and perhaps hospital personnel and the attorney representing the witness. After being sworn in, the attorney who is seeking to discover the witness's information about the event will explain the questioning process and will carefully and specifically request that the witness ask for clarification if a question is not understood. The witness needs to be alert and able to understand all that is being asked. The witness will be asked some preliminary identifying information such as name, address, workplace, work experience, and educational background. (The technologist may want to prepare in advance a curriculum vitae which outlines education and experience; see Appendix for sample form.) The witness may be asked if he or she is currently taking any medications and, if so, to identify the drug. The witness may also be asked if he or she is under the influence of any narcotics or mood-altering drugs.

Such questions are asked to ensure that the witness's mind is clear and focused and that nothing has been taken that might influence the witness's ability to respond to questions. If a request for records was part of the subpoena, the witness will be asked if such documents are present at the deposition. The lawyer will want to know if the witness has discussed the event with anyone. If the witness has discussed the case with an attorney, the witness's attorney may say, "Objection, privileged" and instruct the witness not to answer the question. The two attorneys will then discuss the objection, and the witness may be advised to respond, or another question will be asked. The meat of the deposition as a witness is personal recollections of the event and information from any contemporaneous written or taped documents made at the time of the incident. (See Appendix for a sample deposition taken regarding a radiograph.)

**5.** Once the deposition has been completed, the witness will be advised that he or she may be expected to testify at trial, which may be either before a jury or before a judge without the jury, which is known as a *bench trial*. The attorney, who is calling the witness, has the duty to inform the person and the court that he or she intends to call that individual as a witness. The technologist will again receive a written document, most likely entitled a *summons,* and will be ordered to attend or face legal consequences.

**6.** Until the time of trial, the technologist may be periodically contacted by the attorney who is relying on the witness's testimony, to keep the technologist advised of the current status of the litigation. In some circumstances, the witness may be called upon to complete the deposition or to review the testimony to determine its accuracy before trial.

Most lawsuits are settled during or upon completion of the discovery phase. Presiding judges encourage settlement negotiations by conducting pretrial conferences in advance of the trial, so that preliminary matters can be disposed of and issues can be defined. Pretrial motions, including *motions in limine* which seek to exclude certain evidence from being presented at trial, will be presented at this time. The attorneys will advise the court of the witnesses to be called, and the court will try to accommodate time schedules when setting a trial date.

A lawsuit can be settled at any time during the trial or before, as long as a verdict has not been rendered. Therefore, witnesses may be called to appear, only to be sent home because a settlement has been reached.

## The Trial

Suppose the parties cannot reach a settlement and the case continues to trial. The radiographer who has carried out the physician's order is now set to appear at trial as a witness. Testimony at trial will include evidence of what orders were received and how and in what form they were received. If the orders came by written instruction from the physician, the technologist will be requested to identify the order, testify that it was the one received on the date in question, and answer questions about the order or procedure. The document itself must be admitted into evidence through a specific procedural process carefully followed by the attorney who is seeking the admission. Most states have rules of evidence which guide evidentiary admission or have adopted the Federal Rule of Evidence.[21]

If the radiologic science professional is asked to provide testimony as an expert, the answers to questions asked will be used to instruct the judge or jury about scientific or technical knowledge which will help them better understand the evidence.[22] In order to be permitted to testify as an expert, the radiographer must be qualified. The expert must demonstrate to the court through the answers to specific questions that he or she has the specific knowledge, skills, education, and experience necessary to testify concerning the event in question. Only upon the court's determination of qualification will a witness be asked to state an opinion as to how a specific radiologic procedure should be conducted or what the procedural requirements are for performing an MRI, a sonogram, a nuclear scan[23] or another radiographic procedure.[23]

After both sides have presented their evidence, the judge or jury will render a verdict for the party who has made the most convincing argument based on evidence presented. The decision must be based solely on information presented through sworn testimony. Information brought in from outside may not be used, and the jury should not allow their emotions to lead them to a decision that goes against the weight of the evidence presented.

## CONCLUSION

Being sued or being a witness in a lawsuit is not to be treated lightly. An employee should be familiar with what, if any, protections an employer will provide in the event that the employee is named individually in a lawsuit arising from the performance of employment duties. Will the employer cover legal expenses? Does the employer's liability policy cover employees named individually? Is liability insurance available for your profession? Is it in the best interests of the employee to maintain professional liability coverage? Will the employer's counsel advise the employee and be present at depositions or other fact-finding endeavors?

Employers must be concerned for their employees as well as their organization. Ignoring the concerns of employees may cause them to go elsewhere for assistance or may force them to answer questions from opposing counsel because of intimidation and lack of understanding of the process. An organization may be harmed in a lawsuit if employees are allowed to talk to unauthorized individuals about a particular incident without advice from counsel.

Radiologic science professionals are not now generally named individually in medical negligence lawsuits. As the consumer patient becomes more aware of patients' rights and the responsibilities of individual providers, the incidence of naming individuals may increase. Therefore, it is imperative that professionals have a basic understanding of the law and the role they may play in a lawsuit or other legal action.

## NOTES

1. References to state laws, cases, or other procedural matters will be to the legal system within the Commonwealth of Kentucky, unless otherwise stated.
2. Preamble, *Constitution of the United States.*
3. See "Physicians, Osteopaths and Podiatrists," *Kentucky Revised Statutes* (KRS), ch. 311, KRS 311.571.
4. Idem, KRS 311.572.
5. For a general overview of the adoption of English common law in the United States, see H. Jones, J. Kernockan, and A. Murphy, *Legal Method* (Mineola, NY: Foundation Press, 1980), ch. 7, 737–759.
6. See KRS 413.140(1)(e):
   (1) The following actions shall be commenced within one (1) year after the cause of action accrued: . . .
      (e) An action against a physician, surgeon, dentist or hospital licensed pursuant to KRS Chapter 216, for negligence or malpractice.
7. See Rule 11, Kentucky Rules of Civil Procedure, *Kentucky Rules of Court* (St. Paul: West, 1993). This rule requires that an attorney's signature on a legal document, such as a complaint, "constitutes a certification by him that he has read the pleading, motion or other paper; that to the best of his knowledge, information, and belief formed after reasonable injury, it is well grounded in fact. . . ."
8. Page W. Keeton et al., *Prosser and Keeton on the Law of Torts,* 5th ed. (St. Paul, MN: West, 1984), §32, 187.
9. Deutsch v. Shein, 597 S.W.2d 141 (Ky. S. Ct. 1980).
10. *Black's Law Dictionary,* 5th ed. (St. Paul: West, 1979), 795.
11. See KRS 314, Registered Nurses: Practical Nurses; KRS 314.073, Continuing Education Requirements.
12. *Black's,* 337.
13. Ibid., 223.
14. Ibid., 282.
15. Ibid., 43.
16. Rule 11, Kentucky Rules of Civil Procedure.
17. The discovery phase of a lawsuit is run by specific procedural rules which control the investigatory process. See, for example, Rules 26–37 of the Kentucky Rules of Civil Procedure.
18. See T. L. Osborne and E. T. Osborne, *Trial Handbook for Kentucky Lawyers* (Rochester, NY: Lawyer's Co-Op, 1984), ch. 6–8.
19. See Rule 26.02(1) Kentucky Rules of Civil Procedure.
20. Osborne and Osborne, Trial Handbook, ch. 18.
21. See Ronald W. Eades, *Kentucky Juris Prudence* (Rochester, NY: Lawyers Co-Op, 1987), ch. 1.

22. Edward J. Imwinkelried, *Evidentiary Foundations* (Charlottesville, VA: The Michie Company, Div. of Bobbs-Merrill, 1980).
23. Ibid., ch. 8. (An excellent reference which explains the various procedures attorneys must follow to qualify a witness as an expert, to introduce and authenticate documentary evidence, and to determine the admissibility of various forms of evidence.)

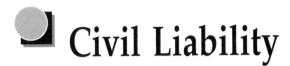

# Civil Liability

Mark Webster

Civil liability covers not only acts that a person intends to commit, but also negligence, which includes acts and consequences that might not have been intended. Both theories arise from a body of law known as torts. A *tort* is a civil wrong in which liability is based on unreasonable conduct. The most famous treatise on torts defines a tort as a "civil wrong, other than breach of contract, for which the court will provide a remedy in the form of an action for damages."[1] In short, if radiologic technologists do something unreasonable in the course of their practice, it could cost them money. This chapter will cover the nature and extent of such financial liability.

Before beginning a discussion of liability, one might reasonably ask how a technologist could be sued. Wouldn't the medical institution that hired the technologist, the doctors who gave the orders, or other medical personnel who supervised the work be ultimately responsible if anything went wrong? Not necessarily. Remember who deals with the patient on the front lines in the imaging or therapy department: the technologist or therapist.

According to one professor of anthropology, "Medicine is a social drama as well as a physical science."[2] In this drama, the technologist or therapist will act as the human link representing the face of medicine to the public. These personnel will greet patients, walk them to the diagnostic center, perform testing, and send them on their way. Since technologists will have the most personal contact with the patient, they may be the most likely to be sued should anything go wrong or should the patient perceive that anything went wrong. The technologist could be sued just as readily as the hospital, the doctor, or the nurse.

Plaintiffs in civil lawsuits seek money damages. In filing a suit, they will sue as many individuals and entities as could conceivably be liable for any wrongs committed. Not only will plaintiffs look for a "deep pocket" for compensation, they will join all the pockets of all persons who have been associated with this case. If a jury makes an award in a trial, it will apportion the award according to who is at fault. Being the low figure on the health care totem pole is no defense. That is why technologists need to know the nature and extent of liability.

## INTENTIONAL TORTS

*Intentional torts* are acts that a person *intends* to commit. These torts are sometimes called "intentional interference with the person." All people have a right to freedom from interference with their person. In return, all people have a duty not to interfere with others. The specific intentional torts covered here will be assault, battery, false imprisonment, intentional infliction of emotional distress, and defamation. It is highly unlikely that a technologist would ever intend to commit one of these torts. But if the patient feels the professional intentionally committed the tort, it will ultimately be up to a jury to decide the intent of the action and the extent of the patient's damages.

According to one expert, "the most common health care problem isn't heart disease, it's miscommunication."[3] Many problems could be lessened or avoided altogether with the proper amount of communication with the patients.

### Assault

One usually thinks of the term *assault* in the criminal sense, in which a person intentionally or wantonly causes physical injury to another person by means of a deadly weapon or a dangerous instrument. *Assault* is usually coupled with the term *battery*. In the sense of civil liability, however, the term *assault* means "acts intending to cause a harmful or offensive contact with the person of the other or a third person, or an imminent apprehension of such a contact, and the other is thereby put in such imminent apprehension."[4]

As can be deduced from the definition, the emphasis here is on possible psychological injury, not physical injury. No touching is required in this tort, only apprehension of the harmful or offensive touch. Some everyday examples of this tort would be a person shaking a fist at another person or a person swinging at another person and missing. Pointing a loaded or unloaded weapon at a person is also a good example of the civil sense of assault. There must be a real apprehension of imminent contact. A mere exchange of words, while unprofessional, would not constitute an assault. Some institutional examples of assault, particularly in a diagnostic imaging setting, might be patients' fears that the therapist or technologist is going to slam an x-ray machine down on them or is about to force them to receive injections or ingest some substance they do not want. Other examples might be threats, particularly to juvenile, senile, or recalcitrant patients, that they will be disciplined somehow if they do not cooperate in the diagnostic process.

Technologists might protest that surely this could not happen in an imaging or therapy department. But remember that patients, particularly those who must undergo an MRI or other sophisticated procedure, enter the department with a great deal of fear and apprehension. According to one psychiatrist, "There's no question that for some people it's [MRI procedure] the most horrible medical procedure they've ever had."[5] In one study, 35 percent of patients undergoing an MRI reported feeling anxious.[6] In another study, more than half of the patients said they should have been better informed, particularly about the noise, the temperature, the degree of confinement, and the duration of the procedure.[7] This study suggested an orientation giving more information to patients and training in relaxation techniques.[8] In yet another study, one in ten patients experienced anxiety severe enough to require that the procedure be halted.[9] The authors of this last study concluded that simply talking to patients will relieve anxiety: "If you explain things to people and take the time to tell them what to expect, they do a lot better than if you don't."[10]

Consider two actions that create apprehension in a patient: haste and lack of preparation. A technologist in a hurry, pushing and pulling machinery in a loud and boisterous manner, could produce fear of contact, particularly in a very young or very old patient. A patient who is not properly prepared for the procedure through conversation with the technologist or through some orientation booklet or film might see all movements as a potential assault. Slow, efficient movements around a patient and a thorough explanation of the physical requirements of the procedure would certainly ease any fear or apprehension that a patient, at least a reasonable patient, might have.

Of course, such torts are not limited to patients. It is possible that technologists could assault each other or that a radiologist could assault a technologist.

Usually the tort of assault will not occur without a resulting battery. Mere emotional disturbance without some sort of injury is not enough to create civil liability for the tort of assault. Likewise, an overly timid or exceedingly nervous patient is not more likely to recover in a lawsuit based on an assault. On the other hand, a stoic, courageous patient should not be any less likely to recover for the tort of assault. Ultimately a jury will decide what is a reasonable apprehension of physical contact. If the jury finds the technologist liable for assault, payment may include money for lost wages, medical treatment, and pain and suffering.

# Battery

The tort of battery will probably be the most common used for recovery against technologists. Technologists are liable to a patient for *battery* if (a) they act "intending to cause a harmful or offensive contact with the person of the other or a third person, or an imminent apprehension of such a contact, and (b) an offensive contact with the person of the other directly or indirectly results."[11]

In short, the tort of battery consists of unwanted contact. The contact has to be more than the occasional bumps and rudeness experienced in everyday activities. A contact is offensive "if it offends a reasonable sense of personal dignity."[12] In short, it is the intention to bring about a contact more offensive than the casual contacts of daily life that is the basis for the tort of battery. A battery could be something originally intended as a practical joke. Just think of people who have been injured as a result of a chair being pulled out from under them. Of course, there is no room for horseplay in the diagnostic imaging or treatment center.

A technologist can be liable for a battery even if the act is intended for the patient's benefit. A technologist who performs a procedure on a patient who has refused to submit to or who has not been properly informed about a procedure will not be relieved of liability for battery even if the technologist believes the procedure would be helpful to the patient.[13] Of course, the key here is to inform the patient properly about the upcoming procedure. Patients should be assessed for the possibility of an anxiety attack. They should be given information about the procedure, the noise, the tight spatial limitations, the temperature, and the duration of the procedure.[14] Many patients do not realize that they do not have to submit to the procedure merely because their doctor has ordered it.

But even the patient who wants to cooperate and submit to the procedure may be frightened by the cold room, the complex machinery, and the various restraints used during the procedure. Pushing or pulling patients to better position them for diagnostic imaging could be a battery. Although restraints will be discussed below with the tort of false imprisonment, the act of restraining a patient, particularly a difficult or immature patient, by use of tape, velcro strips, ropes, collars, or safety belts could constitute a battery.

Since parents can be overprotective of their children and since federal regulations warn radiation workers against continuous exposure to radiation, many hospitals permit the parent, after donning an apron, to hold a child during some procedures, such as an upright x-ray. Parents also may hold their children during other procedures. While this sounds like a foolproof way of avoiding a possible battery against the infant patient, care must be taken not to commit a "double" battery. For example, if the technologist somehow pushes the parent against the child and causes injury to the child, the technologist could be subject to liability to both the parent and the child, should an injury result to one or both. Even if the parent is not injured but the child is, the technologist would still be liable to the child because he or she would be the actor whose act started the chain of events resulting in injury to the child.[15]

In some hospitals, technologists sedate patients before conducting imaging or treatment. The injection itself could be considered a battery if the patient does not want the shot or does not understand that it will be given. Second, even if the patient is asleep, drugged, or anesthetized, a battery could occur. The recipient of the battery does not have to be aware that a battery occurred. For example, there have been cases in which female patients have been abused while sleeping or under anesthetic.[16]

The contact is not limited to touch alone. Any substance that the technologist causes to come into contact with the patient, such as fluids, electric shock, medical instruments, and so on, could constitute a battery. Leaving tape lines on a patient, particularly a child, could be used as evidence that a battery occurred. Likewise, the contact could be with some extension of the patient's body, as in hitting a cane or a walker.

For civil liability to exist, there must be some sort of real injury that can be translated into money damages of the type mentioned in the section on assault. A wrong without damage will not result in liability. Most wrongs, however, do cause damage, ranging from concrete, out-of-pocket expenses to abstract damage for pain and suffering or the loss of services of a spouse or parent.

## False Imprisonment

Closely aligned to the tort of battery is the tort of false imprisonment. On first reflection this sounds slightly ridiculous. How or why would a technologist "imprison" a patient? The basis of the tort is that the patient's right to freedom from confinement is somehow violated. A brief definition of false imprisonment might be "unwanted confinement." According to the legal definition, technologists are subject to liability to a patient for *false imprisonment* if (a) they act "intending to confine the other or a third person within boundaries fixed by the actors, (b) their act directly or indirectly results in such a confinement of the other, and (c) the other is conscious of the confinement or is harmed by it."[17]

The word *confinement* conjures up images of what would happen only in jail. But medical providers also confine patients to small rooms, beds, tables, chairs, and the like. Sometimes, of course, technologists restrain patients for the patients' own good. This tort is somewhat like the tort of assault in that the patient's subjective impression controls whether or not a tort exists. If the patient *feels* confined, then the patient *is*. For example, if a patient believes he or she is locked in a room, even if the room is not locked, the patient could bring a suit for false imprisonment.[18] The tort is unlike the tort of battery in that patients must have some awareness or belief that they are confined. A patient who might have been confined during sleep or while under anesthesia could not sue for false imprisonment. In cases of children or other persons who are not legally competent, this may not be true.

In a hospital setting, patients could think that they were confined if they could not exit the imaging center either because the door was locked or a hospital employee blocked the door. Again, patients should be informed that they have a right to stop a procedure at any time or at any reasonable time during the procedure and that they have a right to leave. In addition, not permitting a patient to communicate with people outside the hospital might constitute false imprisonment.[19]

Probably the most common source of confinement issues will revolve around the use of restraints during testing or treatment involving children. Some diagnostic or treatment centers use no patient restraints; others go to great lengths to restrain patients to ensure a good-quality diagnostic image as well as to prevent injury to the patient and liability on behalf of the medical facility. Some hospitals always restrain infants, while other hospitals see this practice as cruel and unusual.

A quick walk through any imaging center will reveal the instruments of confinement: sandbags, tapes, head sponges, chucks, arm bands, and paper absorbers. No doubt about it: sometimes patients must be confined. Sometimes the use of force to restrain a patient is justified.

As with the other torts, patients might recover damages due to imprisonment if a jury finds the technologist's actions to be unreasonable, unjustified, and unprivileged. The type of damages a patient might receive could be money for "bodily injury, physical discomfort or inconvenience, loss of time and wages, emotional distress, harm to reputation and the loss of the company of one's family."[20] Punitive damages could be awarded if the imprisonment were extremely unreasonable.[21]

## Intentional Infliction of Emotional Distress

A relatively new tort is the intentional infliction of emotional distress, sometimes known as the tort of *outrage*. This chapter will not discuss *negligent* infliction of emotional distress. The tort of *intentional infliction of emotional distress* is defined as follows: "(1) One who by extreme and outrageous conduct intentionally or recklessly causes severe emotional distress to another is subject to liability for such emotional distress, and if bodily harm to the other results from it, for such bodily harm."[22] Another legal treatise lists four elements of this tort: (1) conduct of the defendant was outrageous, (2) the defendant acted intentionally or recklessly; (3) severe emotional distress was suffered by the plaintiff; and (4) the defendant's conduct was the proximate cause of emotional distress suffered.[23]

This tort might have limited applicability to technologists because the conduct would have to be so extremely outrageous that it would be totally unexpected. The conduct in this tort must be so bad that any reasonable person would describe it as outrageous. This is conduct that is "beyond all possible bounds of decency, and to be regarded as atrocious and utterly intolerable in a civilized community."[24] For example, perhaps as a practical joke, a technologist might falsely imply or falsely state to a patient that a certain diagnostic test shows some horrible disease or condition. If this causes the patient to suffer nervous shock and resulting illness, the technologist would be liable to the patient for this illness.[25]

If a technologist threatens to beat up or harm a patient and this causes the patient to become extremely frightened and emotionally distressed, then the technologist could become liable to the patient for any resulting illness. Also, if a technologist ridiculed or embarrassed the patient for some reason, perhaps in a feeble attempt to encourage cooperation, and this caused the patient injury, liability for the intentional infliction of emotional distress might result.

With this tort, the relationship between the parties is assumed to be such that, if one party is responsible for the other or has some apparent authority over the other, the person in authority might more likely be held liable for intentional infliction of emotional distress as a result of the abuse of that position. This tort is most often seen with police officers, school principals, and debt collection agents. Arguably, technologists are also in a position of apparent authority because patients give over, at least symbolically, their bodies for clinical testing and are put in a somewhat vulnerable position. If a technologist for some reason threatens to have the patient arrested or bullies the patient, who then becomes distressed, the technologist might be liable to the patient for any damages or resulting illness.

Even worse is the health professional who takes advantage of a weaker person or someone who is more susceptible to emotional distress. An example of this might be the elderly patient who already suspects the presence of a fatal problem, only to have a technologist make light of it. Rough or flagrant treatment of such an elderly person which causes illness from emotional distress might result in a lawsuit.

It is not enough that the conduct be merely insulting or cause hurt feelings; it has to be outrageous and humiliating. A not very far-fetched example might be one in which a pregnant woman brings her child into the department. If the technologist mistreats the child to such a degree that the mother suffers emotional distress, which induces a miscarriage, then the technologist would be liable for the results of the miscarriage or other illness.[26]

Likewise, comments about a patient's physical problems or deformities could bring about a claim for intentional infliction of emotional distress.

Since grossly obese patients are often more difficult to scan or image, and because the resulting imagery is often not clear, technologists should refrain from making any comments about a patient's obesity.

It is possible to be liable for conduct directed at third parties. This section will not discuss actions by unrelated bystanders recovering from emotional distress caused by the negligence of the defendant. However, the law is growing in this area. This is most often seen when a mother sees her child hit by a car or when anyone sees a tragic accident and in turn is damaged physically or psychologically by the sight.

## Defamation

Closely related to the tort of intentional infliction of emotional distress is the tort of defamation. The very same outrageous conduct that serves as a basis for an action for intentional infliction of emotional distress could support a defamation action.[27] The right protected in the tort of *defamation* is the right to one's good name. Usually this tort is associated with tabloid stories about the private lives of movie stars. The tort of defamation, however, has everyday applications, particularly in the hospital workplace. The tort of defamation has four elements: (a) a false and defamatory statement concerning another; (b) an unprivileged publication to a third party; (c) fault amounting at least to negligence on the part of a publisher; and (d) either actionability of the statement irrespective of special harm or the existence of special harm caused by the publication.[28] Basically this tort consists of telling a lie about someone or putting them in a false light.

The "publication" is a communication made either intentionally or negligently to a third person. There is no defamation when the alleged defamatory remark is made directly and only to the patient. The communication can be either written or spoken. Again, there must be some sort of resulting injury. In this case, the injury is the harm to the reputation of another which results in the lowering of that person's reputation in the community or would result in deterring third persons from associating or dealing with the defamed person.[29]

Libel and slander are two forms of defamation. *Libel* concerns publication of defamatory matter by writing. *Slander* concerns publication of defamatory matter by any other means, most commonly by the spoken word. In the context of the radiologic technologist, defamation could occur in what the technologist says about the patient to a third party, such as a fellow employee, a patient's family member, or a bystander; or in what the technologist writes about the patient, usually in the form of hospital or lab notes. Interestingly, anything can be said about dead people. Deceased persons cannot be defamed.[30] It is possible to defame a group or class, but this division of the tort will not be discussed here because it is unlikely that it would occur in a hospital setting.

The law on defamation is unusual concerning the proof of damages. In the other torts discussed above, damages must be proven. In this tort, sometimes damages do not have to be proven; they are assumed. Some communication requires proof of real injury or damages, while others do not because the communication is so offensive that some kind of injury is presumed from the publication of the defamatory statement itself. This is sometimes called *defamation per se* or *slander per se.* There are four classes of cases that have been deemed to be defamation per se: imputation of (1) a crime; (2) a loathsome disease; (3) business, trade, or professional misdeeds; or (4) unchastity. The burden of proof in cases involving these types of defamatory remarks is less than in other cases of defamation because here the defamer is subject to liability without proof of special harm.[31]

A simple example might explain the difference in the burden of proof. A statement to a third person that a patient is lazy might result in a suit for defamation, but the defamed person would have to prove that he or she was somehow injured by the statement. However, a statement to a third party that a patient has AIDS understandably carries the presumption that it is damaging even if it is false.

The best method of preventing this tort is to be professional at all times, in person and on paper. Extraneous remarks should be omitted. Personal opinions are unimportant. What need not be said must not be said. What place would allegations of criminal activity have in a hospital setting after all? Information about so-called loathsome diseases may have more relevance but should be stated in an objective, clinical way.

It is interesting how the idea of what constitutes a loathsome disease has changed over the years. Recently, this usually referred to venereal diseases. Earlier, it referred to incurable diseases such as leprosy but, interestingly, not to smallpox or tuberculosis.[32] In recent cases, false allegations that a person has AIDS have been held to be defamatory per se. For example, the former boyfriend of a schoolteacher put large signs in public places claiming that she had AIDS. The jury awarded her $100,000.[33] Perhaps mental illness could be considered a loathsome disease, but courts have not been consistent in labeling these types of cases as such or in making awards in these types of cases.

In today's society, it is much more likely that slanderous remarks will concern allegations of sexual activities. The rules in this area originally protected only the rights of women to their virtuous name. However, as society is changing, so is this, and there is no place for allegations of this nature in a hospital setting.

Likewise in the last special area of defamation, the hospital or treatment or diagnostic center is no place for statements that might concern individuals' businesses or professions, particularly their ability to do business honestly. Oddly enough, recent reported incidents of defamation in the hospital setting concern statements made about *physicians* by other hospital personnel.

Although truth is a defense in defamation cases, it might take a trial to determine which version of the truth will prevail. Likewise, one can use the idea of privilege as a defense against a charge of defamation. Privileges can be either absolute, qualified, or conditional. These privileges are almost nonexistent in hospital settings. An example of an absolute privilege would be remarks made by legislators within their legislative function.[34] Likewise, statements made in the pleading of a lawsuit which are relevant to the issues of the suit are sometimes considered absolutely privileged from liability. The common law identified three types of conditional or qualified privileges: (1) conditional privilege arising from an occasion; (2) privileged critics or "fair comment"; and (3) special privileges concerning reports at special proceedings or public meetings.[35] These privileges generally are applicable to the media only and will not be discussed here.

## VICARIOUS LIABILITY

It is possible for someone to be liable for negligence they did not commit. Sometimes the negligence of one person can be *imputed*, or placed upon, another, even if the other is not present. The other person is said to be *vicariously liable* for the action of the actor. For example, in a recent case, a hospital employee bandaged an injured child's finger so tightly that the finger eventually had to be amputated. The mother, who was a nurse, pleaded with a doctor she knew who was in the emergency room to treat her daughter. The doctor, who was not a hospital employee and had no duty to treat the child, performed the necessary treatment and told an emergency room employee to wrap the wound. The kind doctor was sued under the theory that the hospital was working under his direction and was therefore a "borrowed servant."[36]

The most common type of vicarious liability is known as *respondeat superior.* The meaning of this Latin term is almost obvious. A superior may be called upon to respond to the actions of his servant. Briefly, the master may be liable for the acts of the servant. In hospital settings, there are few masters and many servants. For example, a doctor could become liable for the actions of hospital personnel; hospital superiors in an imaging center might become liable for the actions of other department workers. Likewise, if a student technologist caused an x-ray machine to overheat and burn a patient, the hospital and the doctor in charge of the procedure could be liable.[37] The basic idea is that one who orders a thing done by another is acting as if the orderer did it. The supervisor usually has the deeper pocket; therefore, the more financially blessed superiors are given the potential for liability. This makes some sense, in that superiors usually profit by the actions of their inferiors and are better able to purchase insurance and limit risks of potential problems. For example, if a patient needs to be injected with some sort of contrast, doctors could conceivably do so.

It would be to their advantage to have the procedure done because they could thereby make a better diagnosis. Likewise, doctors possibly stand to gain financially by the procedure. Since doctors order others to do it, then perhaps the ultimate liability should be traced back to the doctors who might also benefit from the act financially.

For the theory of *respondeat superior* to work, employment has to exist. Whether or not an employer-employee relationship exists depends on whether or not there is a contract of employment; if not, state laws will determine whether such a relationship exists. Usually, independent contractors are liable for their own acts.

The master/employer can be liable for the acts of the employee even if the employer commands the employee *not* to do something. For example, even if the hospital orders the technologist not to bind or tie down a patient, and he or she does it anyway, both the technologist and the imaging center could be sued for battery and false imprisonment because the employee operated outside the scope of management's orders.

Under the theory known as *"captain of the ship,"* the captain could be liable for the negligence of his charges. The most common example of this occurs in the operating room. The chief surgeon would be the "captain," and any problems that might arise either from his or her own actions or those of all other persons involved in the operation could be imputed to the chief surgeon because he or she is thought to be in control of the operation. Perhaps the same theory could be applied to the head of a diagnostic lab.

Of course, if the employee acts outside the scope of employment, then the employer's liability might not be traced back to the employer. For example, a technologist may play with a child patient to relax the child. If that technologist injures the child during the play, the hospital might not be liable for the injury to the child because the technologist is hired to perform diagnostic imaging, not to play with children. This type of horseplay would be outside the scope of a technologist's job. The technologist would then be liable for all damages.

An employer can even be liable for the so-called emotional torts, discussed earlier. An example might be that the hospital could be liable for damages suffered by a patient who is thrown out of the department for some reason. Perhaps if the act is done in the furtherance of a hospital purpose, the technologist's actions could be imputed to the hospital. But if the conduct is outrageous because it is unusual or unprovoked, the actions of the employee might be imputed to the hospital. (Of course, the hospital might be liable under another theory for hiring such an emotional employee!) Likewise, if an employee misuses equipment or an instrument which is highly dangerous in and of itself and hurts the patient, the harm could be imputed to the hospital on a theory of negligent use of an instrument.

It is unlikely that a technologist will be employed in a joint enterprise, but the law treats joint enterprises the same way as partnerships. Each partner or joint member is the agent of all the others and could be liable for the actions of all the others.

## ELEMENTS OF TORTS

In general, torts are said to have four elements which must be proved in order to win a judgment: (1) duty, (2) breach of duty, (3) damages, and (4) damages proximately caused by the breach. Legal matters are divided into civil cases and criminal cases. As mentioned earlier, this chapter deals only with civil cases, which are cases brought to win money damages. In these cases, the plaintiff or the injured party must prove the case by a preponderance of the evidence. In other words, the plaintiff does not have to prove negligence beyond a reasonable doubt. This burden of proof is substantial but not as great as it is in criminal cases.

Some cases, however, can be proved by circumstantial evidence. What if, after adjusting the collimator of an x-ray machine, a technologist walks back to the booth to begin the x-ray, and the machine falls on top of the patient. Well, "the thing speaks for itself." The technologist has control of the x-ray machine. X-ray machines do not normally collapse on patients. The reasonable conclusion is that, because the technologist was the last one who adjusted the machine, some negligent act on the part of the technologist caused the machine to fall. In effect, the burden of proof shifts to the defendant technologist or hospital to prove that no negligence in fact occurred. This theory of negligence based on circumstantial evidence is known as *res ipsa loquitur,* or literally "the thing speaks for itself." A recent example involved a patient who discovered after surgery that she still had the tip of a surgical instrument in her right leg.[38] The outcome of this case is obvious.

There are usually four conditions that must exist before the doctrine of *res ipsa loquitur* can be applied: (1) the element must be one that ordinarily does not occur in the absence of someone's negligence; (2) it must be caused by an agency or instrumentality within the exclusive control of the defendant; (3) it must not have been due to any voluntary action or contribution on the part of the plaintiff. Later, a fourth condition was added: evidence as to the explanation of the event must be more readily accessible to the defendant than to the plaintiff.[39] A famous application of the *res ipsa loquitur* doctrine in hospital cases occurred in a California hospital. In that case, a patient undergoing an appendectomy suffered traumatic injury to his shoulder, an unusual happening in an abdominal surgery. The doctrine of *res ipsa loquitur* was applied against all the doctors and hospital employees connected with the injury.[40] This is understandable because someone in that group had to have acted negligently to cause a shoulder problem resulting from an appendectomy.

## JURISDICTION

Although most medical professionals may not realize it, they live simultaneously in two kingdoms. They live in a single state and at the same time in the United States. What this means in terms of civil liability is that, in the event of a claim of negligence, the technologist may be sued in state or federal court. Obviously, plaintiffs will try to sue where they are most likely to win. Usually in civil liability cases, the claimant will sue in the location where the injury occurred. This is the easiest choice because obviously a local court would have jurisdiction over a wrong done in its state. Problems arise when an injured person from another state brings a suit in his or her own state. In other words, the defendant ends up being sued in the court of a state he or she has never visited. It is also possible to be sued in a federal court. When a citizen of one state sues a citizen of a different state, this situation is known as *diversity jurisdiction* and vests a federal court with jurisdiction over the case when the matter and controversy exceed the sum or value over $50,000 exclusive of interest or costs. Even if a matter starts in state or federal court, it might be *removed,* or transferred, to a different state or federal court.

## CONCLUSION

Technologists are trained to be competent health professionals, not defendants in lawsuits. Being professional at all times, understanding what is required, understanding the technology, and communicating with patients will help avoid civil liability and keep both technologist and facility out of court.

## N O T E S

1. W. Prosser and R. Keeton, *The Law of Torts,* 5th ed. (St. Paul, Minn.: West Publishing Co., 1985).
2. Bob Kronemeyer, "Both Sides of the Stethoscope," *Notre Dame News,* Summer 1993, pp. 12–13.

3. Kronemeyer, "Both Sides," p. 12.
4. *Restatement (Second) of Torts*, §21 (1977).
5. Miriam Shuchman, "When Noninvasive Scan Causes a Patient's Panic," *New York Times*, 3 November 1993, p. B8.
6. S. C. Brennan, W. H. Redd, P. B. Jacobsen, et al., "Anxiety and Panic During Magnetic Resonance Scans," *Lancet* 1 (1988): 512.
7. M. B. Quirk, A. J. Letendre, R. A. Ciottune, and J. F. Lingley, "Anxiety in Patients Undergoing MRI Imaging," *Radiology* 70 (1989): 464.
8. Quirk et al., "Anxiety," 465.
9. J. C. Melendez and B. McCrank, "Anxiety related reactions associated with magnetic resonance imaging examinations," *Journal of the American Medical Association* 270 (1993): 745–747.
10. Schuchman, "When Noninvasive Scan," p. B8.
11. *Restatement (Second) of Torts*, §13 (1977).
12. *Restatement (Second) of Torts*, §19 (1977).
13. *Restatement (Second) of Torts*, §15 and §20 (1977).
14. Melendez and McCrank, "Anxiety related reactions," 747.
15. *Restatement (Second) of Torts*, §14, Comment b, and §20 (1977).
16. *Restatement (Second) of Torts*, §18, Comment b (1977).
17. *Restatement (Second) of Torts*, §35 (1977).
18. *Restatement (Second) of Torts*, §42, Comment d (1977).
19. Stowers v. Weolodzko, 191 NW2d 355 (1971).
20. L. S. Goldstein and M. J. Zaremski, *Medical and Hospital Negligence* (Deerfield, Ill.: Callaghan, 1990), 35.
21. Dick v. Watonwan County, 562 F.Supp. 1083 (D. Minn. 1983), rev'd other grounds, 738 F2nd 939 (8th Cir. 1989).
22. *Restatement (Second) of Torts*, §46(1) (1977).
23. *Shepard's Causes of Action* (Colorado Springs: Shepard's McGraw-Hill, 1983), vol. 7, 663.
24. *Restatement (Second) of Torts*, §46, Comment d (1977).
25. *Restatement (Second) of Torts*, §46 (1977)
26. *Restatement (Second) of Torts*, §46 (1977).
27. Campos v. Oldsmobile, Div., GM Corp., 246 NW2d 352 (1976); Dazzo v. Meyers, 443 NYS2d 245 (1981).
28. *Restatement (Second) of Torts*, §558 (1977).
29. *Restatement (Second) of Torts*, §559 (1977).
30. *Restatement (Second) of Torts*, §560 (1977).
31. *Prosser and Keeton, Law of Torts*, 778.
32. S. Speiser, C. F. Krause, and A. W. Gans, *The American Law of Torts* (New York: Clark, Boardman, Callaghan, 1991), 29.65.
33. Snipes v. Mack, 381 SE2d 318 (1989).
34. *Restatement (Second) of Torts*, §590, Comment 9 (1977).
35. *Restatement (Second) of Torts*, §590 (1977).
36. Lighterman v. Porter, 548 S2d 891 (Fla. App. 1989).
37. Barber v. St. Frances Cabrini Hospital, Inc., 345 So2d 1307 (La. 1977).
38. Gravitt v. Newman, 495 NYS2d 439 (1993).
39. Prosser and Keeton, *Law of Torts*, 244.
40. Ybarra v. Spangard, 208 P2d 445 (1949).

# Medical Negligence and Malpractice

J. Thomas Galle

There are many variables in the concepts of medical negligence and malpractice. The purpose of this chapter is to acquaint the reader with some of the familiar and perhaps not so familiar concepts. The particular cases used are generally within the author's jurisdiction, but the overall issues are fairly consistent in other jurisdictions. It is always a good idea to learn the basic rule in the practitioner's own local jurisdiction.

One of the first concepts in this area is the general idea of negligence. The 1990 edition of *Webster's Illustrated Dictionary* defines *negligence* as:

1. **The state or quality of being negligent.**
2. **Any negligent act or failure to act.**
3. **The omission or neglect of any reasonable precaution, care, or action, resulting in accident, injury or loss.**[1]

*Black's Law Dictionary* defines *negligence* as:

**The omission to do something which a reasonable man, guided by those ordinary considerations which ordinarily regulate human affairs, would do, or the doing of something which a reasonable and prudent man would not do. . . .**
**The law of negligence is founded on reasonable conduct under all circumstances of (a) particular case. Doctrine of negligence rests on duty of every person to exercise due care in his conduct toward others from which injury may result.**[2]

The former definition states simply that an action occurs but does not go much further regarding the consequences of such actions or omissions. The legal concept in the latter definition considers the results of an action (or an omission). The latter definition is what will be briefly explored here.

## NEGLIGENCE

The legal concept of negligence necessarily involves three steps. The first step involves that which regulates human behavior toward others. This means essentially what duties are owed to others. If an action is required, for example, then there is a duty to perform that action in a reasonable and prudent manner. Failure to act reasonably and prudently could be considered negligence. Acting in a manner inconsistent with accepted norms could also be considered negligence.

If a patient is brought to the radiology department, the responsibility for that patient's well-being passes to the radiographers and any other personnel assigned to the department or patient. It is their duty to see that the procedures performed follow the accepted guidelines. A failure to follow these norms of practice could constitute negligence. If a procedure calls for restraints to be used, to prevent a fall or to prevent harm to the patient or others, the need to restrain should be explained and the restraints should be properly applied. Failure to properly apply restraints could result in injury to the patient or others, for which the radiographer and the facility may be liable.

There has been a great deal of discussion and case law over the years involving just what is "reasonable," and, suffice it to say, the general meaning is its everyday, common-sense definition. If an action falls outside the bounds of common sense, chances are that it will fit the definition of negligence. The rule of thumb is to decide whether the action makes sense. If it doesn't, it shouldn't be done. Of course, there are many exceptions to this rule, but the concept is grounded in the fact that humans are rational creatures capable of making rational decisions.

The second step necessarily involved in the issue of negligence is failure or breach of the duty owed to the individual. Once duty to the individual is established, the actor has the obligation to perform that duty in a manner that will bring it to a successful conclusion. If the actor fails in that duty, he or she may be responsible to the individual to whom that duty was owed for any injury resulting from that failure.

This brings us to the third and final step in the concept of negligence. This step involves damage to the individual for breach of duty. For the legal concept of negligence to apply, there must be some damage to the person or property resulting from breach of the duty owed. If the patient falls because of improper restraint or monitoring and suffers a fractured cervical spine, for example, the damages could be enormous. On the other hand, that same fall could result in no injury. Other than an apology and an appropriate review of the situation, no damages could accrue. There would be no additional medical expense or other nonspecific damages. If there is no damage, then, under the legal definition, there may be no negligence.

There are also notions of *nominal damages,* which indicate a willingness to find someone at fault and that there is a consequence for acting in a negligent manner. There are those cases in which very small or nominal damages are awarded. These types of cases are brought because of the principle involved. This could be a legal point which may need clarification, or it may be simply one's dedication to a cause which needs to be defined in a court of law. If, in the noninjury fall, for example, there is found to be a complete disregard for the patient's well-being, that negligence might be utilized to effect a change in the procedure or attitude of the institution. There may not be a great deal of money at stake, but the principle may be the key motivating factor.

The entire legal system in the negligence arena has developed through years of cases attempting to define this concept, and it will continue to evolve. Depending on one's point of view, the system may be for the better or for the worse. In any event, it will continue to undergo change and refinement. It is imperative for professionals to keep up with major changes in this area, and changes that affect professional practice should be updated regularly through proper channels of communication.

Before *medical* negligence can be discussed, there are two further areas of negligence which need to be explored. These two concepts, depending on the jurisdiction, are important to know because of the legal and financial consequences of each.

## Contributory Negligence

As the principle of negligence evolved, it was considered that, for a party to recover, he or she should be free of any negligence. It was felt that a party making a claim for damages should not have contributed to his or her own injury and then recover for it. This doctrine of negligence became known as *contributory negligence.*

Thus, if the injured party shared the blame in an accident, recovery is denied. This concept itself has undergone many refinements, and several exceptions have arisen in order to get around being completely barred. In many jurisdictions, the concept of *slight versus gross* has become the accepted practice. This concept is basically what it says. If the contributory negligence is "slight," or minimal, recovery can be had. Conversely, if the contributory negligence is considered "gross," then the grounds exist for no recovery.

The above concept has worked as a practical matter, but still involves making judgments regarding liability. Juries have been asked to determine whether the contributory negligence of the plaintiff was sufficient to deny recovery. The most common examples of contributory negligence barring recovery are in cases of slipping and falling. The reported cases are too numerous to cite, but the overriding principle in many cases was the argument that the plaintiff should have been looking, or should have known of a step, or should have seen the carton in the aisle. Many juries denied recovery because they felt the plaintiff should have been aware of where they were going and that their contributory negligence was sufficient to deny all recovery. This concept was the majority rule for many years.

There was one exception to this rule which developed as a way of recovering in spite of contributory negligence. This doctrine became known as the *last clear chance* doctrine. Essentially, this doctrine means that the plaintiff can still recover damages if, while in a position of peril, the defendant had the last clear chance to avoid the accident. An obvious example of this doctrine is the case of a plaintiff who is hit by a car. If that plaintiff is found to be contributorily negligent for crossing against the light, he or she may not recover damages. However, the plaintiff may still recover if it can be shown that the defendant was a block away and had plenty of time to slow down or stop. This means that the defendant had the "last clear chance" to avoid the accident but failed to do so.

## Comparative Negligence

Many jurisdictions have felt that there was something inherently wrong with a doctrine of negligence that completely barred recovery for damages because of negligence by both parties. There should be a way to lessen the burden and still maintain judicial fairness. From this concern arose the second doctrine of negligence, known as *comparative negligence.*

Comparative negligence developed because there was a need to address the apparent inequities in denying recovery for shared fault. Many jurisdictions felt that this resulted in a windfall for either the plaintiff or the defendant, depending on the degree of fault found and against which party.

The courts and legislatures then embarked on a quest to define this new doctrine. Comparative negligence developed into two basic forms: pure and modified. *Modified comparative negligence* depends on the degree of fault, but recovery may be barred if the degree of fault is high enough.

Recovery under the modified comparative fault system may be barred completely if the plaintiff's negligence is equal to the defendant's fault. This is sometimes referred to as the *50 percent rule.* Under this theory, a plaintiff's recovery diminishes proportionally to his or her degree of fault. When fault is considered equal (50/50), both parties can recover 50 percent of damages, but once the degree of fault exceeds 50 percent, there is no recovery for the plaintiff.

Another version holds that the plaintiff's fault must be "less than" that of the defendant. This is sometimes called the 49 percent rule. As long as the plaintiff was less negligent than the defendant, recovery is allowed. Thus, a 50/50 case could result in no recovery.

*Pure comparative negligence,* on the other hand, means just that: pure. Each party shares the blame to the degree to which he or she contributed to the accident. There is no cut-off point that completely bars recovery. Theoretically, it is possible to collect 1 percent of the plaintiff's damages if the defendant is deemed 1 percent negligent.

The watershed case in Kentucky, *Hilen v. Hayes,* is a concise history of the doctrine of negligence.[3] The facts of this case show the inequities in applying contributory negligence as a complete bar to recovery. Ms. Hilen was severely injured in an automobile accident. There was no doubt that the fault for the collision was that of the driver of the car in which she was a passenger. The defendant argued, however, that Ms. Hilen was contributorily negligent because she failed to exercise reasonable care by riding with a person whom she knew or should have known was too intoxicated to drive. The jury found that Ms. Hilen was contributorily negligent and barred her completely from recovering any of her damages.

The Kentucky Supreme Court found that this system was not fair and determined that comparative negligence would apply. The court went further, to state that the form of comparative negligence in Kentucky would be the "pure" form.

Under this form, and given the same facts as above, the jury could determine the total damages and the degree of the plaintiff's fault. The recovery in that instance would be the total amount reduced by the degree of fault. A case worth a total of $100,000 with the plaintiff 25 percent at fault would result in a $75,000 recovery, for example.

It should be kept in mind that the defendant can recover damages as well. If the plaintiff's negligence played a part in damaging the defendant, the defendant can collect his or her pro-rata share.

## MEDICAL NEGLIGENCE

All of the concepts in negligence apply to medical negligence as well. There is another step involved, however: there must be a relationship between the provider and the patient giving rise to the duty owed. The general rule is that, when one sees a doctor for a particular condition or examination and the physician agrees to perform the necessary services, the implication is that the physician will render those services with requisite skill and care. This service is rendered in exchange for the payment of the normal charges for providing this care.[4] The physician's failure to provide those services with that requisite skill and care gives rise to action in medical negligence.[5]

## Element of Duty

Once the relationship is established, there is a duty to use that degree of care and skill expected of a reasonably competent practitioner in the same class to which the physician belongs, acting in the same manner and under similar circumstances.[6] Thus, the medical professional is expected to perform his or her duty to the patient according to the standards in the field in which the medical professional practices. A "reasonably competent" practitioner is one who should, at a minimum, know the basics in treating a patient. The same is true in related fields. There are professional standards in all areas of health care, and diagnostic imaging and radiation therapy are no exception. Those standards are to be followed, and the practitioner may be accountable for any deviation from them.

This represents a departure, to some degree, from previous standards. Although the concept is consistent with past standards, it eliminates the geographical reference. Decisions in the past usually included a statement to the effect that the degree of skill and care was confined to the locality, largely because information was not readily available in all areas. Now that communications have vastly improved, information is readily available, almost at the touch of a computer key.

The courts have been somewhat slow in picking up on this, but they are coming to recognize that advances in medical science and the means of communicating these findings have improved to the point where standards are basically national in nature. Accepted principles of practice are available in various professional publications, and changes wrought by advances and new discoveries are seen everywhere from newspaper articles to television programs. A rural area is just as capable of keeping up with these advances as a large metropolitan area.

## Element of Breach

What, then, constitutes a breach of this duty owed to the patient? That breach occurs when the conduct drops below the ordinarily recognized standard of care for that particular treatment.

This does not mean, however, that an error of judgment on the part of the physician will result in liability. A physician who conducts his or her treatment within the accepted medical practice, but who nonetheless has a bad result, will not be held liable.[7] The courts recognize that medical science is not exact and that not every result will be favorable. Sometimes, even within accepted standards, judgment calls must be made. These judgment calls will not always turn out right.

## Element of Injury

Everyone understands that medical negligence occurs when the wrong limb is amputated or when the improper medication has been prescribed after it was known to be harmful. This brings us to the area of injury and damage.

In the first case, it is easy to see that the injury was inflicted because of malpractice. The patient has been wrongfully injured due to failure to follow accepted standards of practice. The wrong instructions were given, or the right instructions were not followed. Regardless, it is obvious that the patient was injured as a direct result of this negligence. It is also easy to see that the patient has suffered damage as a result of this action. The damage includes not only the immediate effect of the loss of the limb and its attendant medical bills and treatment, it also includes potential loss of earning capacity and pain and suffering. If the behavior was outrageous, then punitive damages may be added to the other damages.

The second case may seem obvious at first, but it lends itself to several areas of discussion. The first and most obvious scenario is one that results in serious injury or death. If this is the case, then the outcome is very similar to that in the first case. There was a duty of prescribing the right medication, a duty of providing the right medication, a breach of that duty, a direct causal relationship between the taking of the wrong medicine, and the injury and loss resulting from the wrong medication. This would meet the criteria for bringing an action for medical negligence.

However, if any of these criteria are missing, then the chances of bringing a medical negligence case are reduced substantially. If there was no duty to prescribe or provide the medication, then there can be no breach of that duty. In this case, there may still be a breach, since medication was given.

If the medication does not cause the injury, there is no actionable case. This is so, even if it was the wrong medication. If there was no injury as a result of the breach, there are no damages to recover under a negligence theory. There may, however, be other legal causes of action available to the plaintiff.

## Burden of Proof

What then, does the party have to show, and how can it be shown? In our legal system, the burden of proof is on the party making the charge. This burden never changes. The party making the allegations must prove, in a civil court, all of the elements described above.

This evidence must be reliable and probative. Reliable and probative evidence is that which can be depended upon and which goes to prove the matter at hand. If it is neither, then it cannot be used.

The Kentucky Supreme Court stated in 1982 that

> In medical malpractice cases the plaintiff must prove that the treatment given was below the degree and skill expected of a reasonably competent practitioner and that the negligence proximately caused the injury or death. . . . The bare possibility of causation will not suffice.[8]

As this finding shows, there must be, again, a deviation from the standard of care *and* this deviation must be the proximate cause of the injury or death. There cannot be one without the other.

The courts have been straightforward as to how this is to be shown by the plaintiff. In these types of actions, the opinions of experts are not only needed, they are required. In most medical negligence cases, proof of causation requires testimony of an expert witness, because the nature of the inquiry is such that jurors are not competent to draw their own conclusions from the evidence without the aid of such expert testimony.[9]

The court repeated the basic exception to that rule in a footnote:

> As an exception to the general rule, expert testimony is not necessary "where the common knowledge or experience of laymen is extensive enough to recognize or infer negligence from the facts."[10]

## Res Ipsa Loquitur

The previously stated case reiterated the fact that the doctrine of *res ipsa loquitur* may be applicable to those situations where the particular injury is of the kind that could be reasonably found would not occur in the absence of negligence. This simply means that the injury could not have occurred unless there was negligence.

An example of this would be a patient who is burned by hot packs while being prepared for surgery. These hot packs are designed to warm the patient but must be removed. If they are not removed, a burn results. Since the patient is semiconscious or unconscious, the only explanation for the result is failure to properly monitor the patient. This is a simple example but nevertheless illustrates the point.

The same analogy could be drawn with the anesthetized or sedated patient in the radiology department. If that patient has not been properly restrained or monitored (if required by policy and the circumstances) and suffers an injury, and there is no plausible way to explain the injury other than negligence on the part of the department personnel, the principle of *res ipsa loquitur* would preclude a defense. The radiographer was negligent, the patient was injured, case closed.

The general rule is that expert medical testimony is required to establish that the standard of care was below accepted practice and that the breach of this standard of care was the proximate cause of injury or death. Other cases may not warrant expert testimony as it may be clear to a layperson, after presentation of the facts, that a breach occurred.

In the fields of diagnostic imaging and therapeutic sciences, there may be some latitude in the area of expert testimony. If the injury occurs from substandard care, expert testimony regarding the standard of care may be required. Were restraints required, and what is the appropriate method for application? Other cases may not warrant expert testimony. Such cases may be as simple as whether negligence can be found for failure to keep the floor clear of materials over which a patient trips, falls, and suffers injury.

## STANDARD OF CARE

That physicians and other professionals are held to a higher standard is a fact of the legal world. In the area of medicine and its related fields, the impression is that there is substantial training and expertise involved in obtaining a degree or certification. Professional organizations have developed particular standards of practice which evolve over time. If the practitioner violates these standards and causes harm or injury, there is the potential for a claim of negligence.

There are guidelines for the procedures to be used by many of the associated fields in medicine. There are guidelines written for hospitals. There are professional standards for medical technology, radiologic sciences, nursing, and other health-related fields. All individuals educated in these fields are expected to know the procedures and guidelines of their respective fields. They are expected to maintain a working knowledge of the advancements made in their fields. When these standards are violated, these individuals may be held accountable for their actions and the consequences of these actions.

One other point which must be made at this juncture is that the courts have held as recently as 1989 that the administration of medical care is a ministerial function and not a discretionary one. This means that employees of a state-owned or -operated medical facility will not be protected under the principle of sovereign immunity.[11]

*Sovereign immunity*, in simple terms, means that government entities or their employees are not susceptible to suit when they are acting in their official capacities. There are many exceptions to this rule, and although these concepts will not be covered here, it is important for individuals working in these types of facilities to understand special liability issues which apply to the performance of their professional practice.

Thus far, this discussion has been confined primarily to physicians, because the majority of cases involve the physician-patient relationship. However, as mentioned previously, there are standards to which other professionals are held. These may be in conjunction with the treating physician or completely independent of the physician's actions.

As an employee of a hospital or other care provider, the individual must maintain the degree of care required for that particular profession. If there is a deviation from that standard of care, which results in injury to the patient, there is exposure to liability.

## *RESPONDEAT SUPERIOR* AND PERSONAL LIABILITY

The general rule is that the employer is responsible for the damages if the employee was acting in the course and scope of his or her employment. The negligence is imputed to the employer through a legal principle known as *respondeat superior*.

What is not generally known is that there is another principle known as *indemnity*, which the employer can use to obtain restitution from the employee for any damages it may have to pay. Most of the time it is not used, but it is a recognized principle. There is the exposure to an employee on a personal basis for damages paid by the employer due to the employee's negligence.

Practically speaking, the application of these concepts of negligence to the diagnostic imaging and therapeutic science professions is essentially the same. These professionals have a duty to perform on behalf of the patient. There are recognized standards of care promulgated for the accepted practice in each field. These standards continue to be updated, and it is the technologist's or therapist's duty to keep informed. Failure to keep up with change can expose a professional to unwanted and expensive legal problems.

As has been pointed out in the previous discussion of negligence in general, there is no longer the complete defense, in many jurisdictions, of claiming that the patient was contributorily negligent. It may reduce the damages assessed, but it will not let a defendant off the hook. In fact, this concept may allow the plaintiff to pull in as many potential defendants as possible. This reduces the plaintiff's share of liability when it can be shown that other players are at fault. It no longer is a doctor-patient lawsuit. It becomes doctor-nurse-technologist-technician-therapist-orderly-and-anyone-else-who-participated-in-the-patient-care-and-subsequent lawsuit.

## CONCLUSION

As an attorney, I have had occasion to interview many individuals regarding potential medical negligence cases. There were those cases that, in my opinion, warranted further action. There were also many cases where lack of communication between the parties gave rise to the suspicion that something was wrong, whereas in reality it was not. Thus, it appears that many potential cases could be avoided through proper communication.

Many strides have been taken in medicine, and there is the perception that almost anything can be done. When an individual is sick, he or she wants to get well. The patient is frightened and confused. If the professional takes the time to talk *with* the patient and not *to* the patient, the patient's fears and suspicions may be lessened. If the professional takes the time to *listen* to the patient and not just *hear* the patient, many potential conflicts may be avoided.

The courts have also spoken to this issue of communication. Although they have addressed it in terms of the physician's legal obligation to fully inform the patient, it also means that this communication must be done at the professional's peril.

> **The relationship of a patient to his physician is by its very nature one of the most intimate. Its foundation is that the physician is learned, skilled and experienced in the afflictions of the body about which the patient ordinarily knows little or nothing but which are of the most importance to him. Therefore, the patient must place great reliance, faith and confidence in the professional word, advice and acts of his doctor. It is the physician's duty to act with the utmost good faith and to speak fairly and truthfully at the peril of being held liable for damages for fraud and deceit.[12]**

The age-old saying that a job worth doing is worth doing well applies especially in the health field. It is the duty of the health care professional to learn his or her skill well, to keep abreast of changes and advancements in knowledge and technology, and to develop the ability to communicate on both a professional and a personal level. There is always the chance that mistakes will occur. The ability to face a mistake and learn from it serves to prevent it from happening again. However, if the professional keeps the patient's well-being in the forefront, the chances of mistakes will be minimized and, if one occurs, the harm may be lessened.

## N O T E S

1. *Webster's Illustrated Dictionary* (1990).
2. *Black's Law Dictionary* (St. Paul: West, 1979).
3. Hilen v. Hayes, 673 S.W.2d 713 (Ky. 1984).
4. Cirafici v. Goffen, 407 N.E.2d 633 (Ill. App. 1980).
5. Ibid.
6. Mitchell v. Hadl, 816 S.W. 2d 183 (Ky. 1991).

7. Holten v. Pfingst, 534 S.W.2d 786 (Ky. 1975).
8. Reams v. Stutler, 642 S.W.2d 586, 588 (1982).
9. Bayless v. Lourdes Hospital, Inc., 805 S.W.2d 122 (Ky. 1991).
10. Ibid., 124.
11. Blue v. Pursell, 793 S.W.2d 823 (Ky. App. 1989).
12. Adams v. Ison, 294 S.W.2d 791, 793–794 (Ky. 1952).

CHAPTER

# 6

 # Documentation and Record Keeping

Ann M. Obergfell

The questions most often asked in the health care arena which are still the hardest to answer are in the area of documentation. What should be documented? How should it be documented? Who should document? Where should information be documented? Why should it be documented? Documentation, like many other areas involving legal issues, will be contingent on state statutes, regulations, and institutional prerogative. There are no clear-cut rules for documentation, but there are fundamental principles that may be used as guidelines when setting up a documentation protocol.

## MEDICAL RECORDS

Medical record keeping is one of the most critical areas of health care and patient management. While some view the voluminous record-keeping requirements as important, primarily for the purpose of medical malpractice defense, there are really many valid reasons for maintaining quality patient care records. The three most recognized reasons for compiling and maintaining the medical record are: (1) documenting the diagnosis, treatment, and progress of the patient; (2) maintaining records for business purposes; and (3) using the records as legal documents.

Documenting the history, diagnosis, treatment plan, and progress of the patient is the most important reason for obtaining an accurate patient medical record. Quality patient care is contingent on the ability of all health care providers to render care based on accurate and timely assessment. The continuity of this care can be maintained only if all individuals providing care are able to document and follow the patient's progress through the records.

A second rationale for keeping documentation of patient treatment is for business purposes. As a business record, the contents can be used to monitor the quality of care the facility has provided to the patient. The Joint Commission on the Accreditation of Health Care Organizations (JCAHO) requires its accredited facilities to set up continuous quality improvement programs. The medical record becomes a part of this program and thus plays a role in the operation of the business. The facility may use the record to ascertain staffing needs, workloads, and utilization of resources. The record is also used to determine reimbursement amounts by agencies such as Medicaid, Medicare, and other third-party payers, such as insurance companies.

Legally, a medical record may be used to benefit the patient, the provider, or the facility. The patient may need the records in an administrative hearing for determining disability and issues of liability, such as worker's compensation or failure of the health care facility to meet the required standard of care in the course of treatment. On the other hand, the individual health care provider or the institution may use the record to demonstrate that the care rendered the patient was within the acceptable standard of care required by law.

Whatever the reason, maintenance of a medical record is an integral part of the health care delivery system. Therefore, every person who enters data, follows a care plan, or reviews the record must understand the importance of keeping a record accurate, objective, and complete.

## REQUIRED DOCUMENTATION

Documentation of patient care varies with the special needs of each facility, but many state laws mandate the minimum requirements for medical records. While the demands on record keeping vary from state to state, certain information is necessary for any patient record. Important data for inpatient facilities include relevant patient history, admitting diagnosis, progress notes, physical examination, diagnostic testing results, and discharge summaries.

Outpatient clinics or centers will require different documentation but still must maintain an accurate and complete record of outpatient services so that continuous quality care can be delivered by all health care providers.

## JCAHO ACCREDITATION RECORD REQUIREMENTS

Facilities accredited by the Joint Commission on the Accreditation of Health Care Organizations are required to maintain certain records on all patients. This information includes name, social security number, medical history, physical examination, physician and other provider treatment order, appropriate informed consent documentation based on facility policy and jurisdictional law, progress notes, reports and results of examinations, surgical and nonsurgical procedures, and discharge summary.[1]

Not all facilities are JCAHO-accredited organizations, but the outline requirements, described in the manual for hospitals, are an excellent guideline for all health care facilities and, with modification for the individual site, would be a reasonable method for determining what records to require and maintain. When state laws do not mandate the information to be included in the record, the courts may use accreditation requirements as a basis for establishing the standard of care.

## DIAGNOSTIC IMAGING SERVICES

Documenting patient care in diagnostic imaging departments has been an area of concern for many years. Although the interpretation report by the radiologist or other qualified physician has always been part of the patient's record, the documentation of care rendered to the patient while in the imaging department has not been clearly defined. Therefore, it is more difficult to determine what information should be entered in the patient record as part of diagnosis and continuity of care.

### Critical Documentation

The most critical question asked about documentation is the one which addresses the type of information to be incorporated in the record. The easy answer is anything which affects the patient's diagnosis and treatment. While this is basically true there are many other pieces of information which will affect the continuity of care and should therefore be included in the record. Sufficient information to justify the diagnosis and warrant the treatment and results is not enough to provide proper care and minimize potential litigation losses.

Critical areas of documentation in medical imaging and therapy include: pertinent patient history, including vital signs; technical variables; contrast media or radiopharmaceutical administration information; pre- and postprocedure directions; names and credentials for personnel involved in the procedure; and the interpretation report by the radiologist or other physician.

## Pertinent Patient History

The foundation of diagnostic imaging and therapy is the patient's history. Procedures and treatments are not performed unless the patient manifests some symptom that brings him or her to a physician or other health care provider. Generally, departmental protocols are designed around patient condition. For example, the protocol for a cervical spine on a trauma patient requires a cross-table lateral cervical that demonstrates all seven cervical vertebrae.[2] This film should be evaluated before the rest of the cervical study and any other procedures are completed.

If the technologist does not know or obtain the pertinent patient history, the procedure may not be completed in an appropriate fashion and according to the standard established by the health care facility and the profession. Relying on an admitting diagnosis may not be sufficient, as this diagnosis may not have any bearing on the procedure that has been ordered. A person may enter the facility for one problem, but another problem may arise during the admission. Likewise, an admitting history of motor vehicle accident (MVA) gives little if any insight into the patient's condition.

Quality interpretation of finished procedures requires that the physician know the pertinent patient history in order to correctly analyze the image and make a diagnosis.[3] The radiologist needs to know the patient's symptoms in order to assess the completed radiographic images while focusing on the suspected area of interest. Also, certain symptoms may encourage a radiologist to look for certain pathological signs or to interpret certain findings differently based on the patient's history.

The JCAHO regulations require that pertinent history be taken on all patients. Therefore, it is the administrator's responsibility to see that this process is part of the department protocol and that all personnel meet the requirements of the process by asking questions and completing the appropriate paperwork.

The department policy should include a standard procedure and a medical history form which will remain with the patient's chart or radiographs. The form used by the department should be designed to direct the flow of questions asked by the technologist and make it easy to complete and incorporate them into the patient record (see Appendix).

## Patient History Form

The form developed by the facility should contain basic information about the patient, such as name, age, gender, birth date, patient identification number, and any other information that will help the technologist ascertain that the right patient receives the ordered procedures. This information can also be used to match the patient with other verifying data.

The form should include places for a female patient's responses to questions concerning pregnancy and last menstrual period (LMP). Some recommend that, for every female patient of childbearing age, a signed form verifying that the patient was informed of the risks associated with radiation exposure during fetal development be attached to the history. This information is documented for two reasons: (1) to protect the patient and fetus from any unnecessary radiation exposure risks and (2) to demonstrate in writing that the technologist followed the acceptable standard for asking and receiving information from the patient. If the answers to the questions concerning pregnancy are not documented and the patient later tests positive for pregnancy, there is no evidence that the technologist offered the necessary information to the patient or asked the appropriate questions.

The form may utilize anatomical drawings which can be marked to show areas of injury or pain. If the department elects to utilize a form with anatomical drawings, the pictures can be used to gain information from patients who may not be able to articulate where they feel pain but can point to the appropriate area on the picture.

The history form should also include a comment section where the technologist or radiologist can write notes concerning the patient or the procedure. Any written information should be objective and factual, utilizing accepted medical terminology and abbreviations.

## *Technical Variables*

The technical variables utilized by the technologists and therapists in the course of testing and treatment should be included in the patient record. The technical information can be part of the record kept in the department with the images, or it can be incorporated into the patient's full record. The technical variables documented by the radiographer should include the number of films taken, the exposure variables (kVp, milliamperage, and time), and if applicable, the amount of fluoro time utilized during the procedure.

Maintaining records of exposure factors can assist other technologists if followup or comparison films are ordered. Patients who are admitted to a facility for an extended period or who are being followed up by a physician will need films on a regular basis. If the technologist can use the technical data supplied by the person who performed the film previously, comparable radiographs can be achieved and the physician will be able to follow the patient's progress. The data can also be used if for some reason it is necessary to calculate the exposure to a given patient. For example, if a patient undergoes an imaging procedure and than discovers that she is pregnant, it will be important to calculate the radiation dose to the fetus. The information generated from these calculations can be utilized when counseling the patient.

## Contrast Media or Radiopharmaceutical Administration

Any time a pharmaceutical is given to a patient, the following informa-tion should be documented: the name of the pharmaceutical adminis-tered, the amount administered, the time of administration, the path or mode of administration, and the name of the person who administered the pharmaceutical.

Contrast media and radioactive isotopes are pharmaceuticals and should therefore be treated in the same fashion as other medications. All pharmaceuticals dispensed to the patient on a nursing floor are docu-mented in the patient record; it is thus imperative that pharmaceuticals given to a patient in the diagnostic imaging department also be charted. These records are important if the patient has a reaction to the contrast or if another pharmaceutical is to be given and a provider needs to check on possible contraindications.

A question arises as to whether the administration of barium should be included in the patient's record. Barium is a foreign substance ingested or administered to a patient, and since complications, although rare, have been reported, it is important that the same recording procedure used for other contrast media be used for barium.

## Pre- and Postprocedure Directions

Some diagnostic procedures require that the patient be appropriately prepared before undergoing a procedure.[4] Notations concerning special diets or other orders should be included in the patient's chart. If these orders are not placed in the chart, other health care providers will not be able to render the appropriate care for the patient and may cause the procedure to be delayed or repeated.

Postprocedure orders are critical for patient safety and well-being. Therefore, it is important that such directives be included in the patient's chart and followed by all health care providers.[5]

## DOCUMENTATION ERRORS AND OTHER PROBLEMS

As has been shown, the medical record is not only a record of the pa-tient's diagnosis, treatment, and progress, it is also a business and legal record. These three purposes are so important that errors in a patient record may lead to serious problems for the patient, the caregiver, and the facility. Many documentation errors are due to simple human error, such as illegible writing of notes, failure to appropriately identify the pa-tient and the record, and use of poor spelling, grammar, and unauthorized abbreviations. Other charting problems include failing to place the correct time of the exam or treatment, failure to correct known charting errors in the prescribed manner, and charting by skipping lines between entries.

These problems can be corrected easily by educating all individuals authorized to chart information in patient records. An educational program should define the charting style that is recognized by the facility. Each health organization should have a facilitywide system of charting. A common system ensures that each health care provider understands the notation and can follow the course of treatment. If each department were to do something different, continuity of care would be lost.

Accepted abbreviations must be adopted by the facility. Using abbreviations that are consistent throughout the system makes for easier understanding of the patient's treatment and progress. Use of abbreviations that are not accepted by the facility may make extra work for a health care provider trying to figure out the abbreviation or, worse, to guess at the meaning or completely ignore the notation.

A list of accepted abbreviations should be easily accessible to any individual who is required to document information in a patient chart or who must review a patient chart to verify orders or other patient data.

Writing in medical records should be legible enough that another individual does not have to guess at what is written. The primary patient complaint concerning the following of written orders is that they cannot decipher handwriting. Inability to read a record may lead to improper or incorrect examination or treatment. In legal proceedings, the health care provider will be better served if those reviewing the records are able to read the entries and determine what was done to or for the patient.

## Correction of Error in the Record

Correcting an error or oversight in a medical record can be deadly in a medical negligence case if the judge or jury believes that the changes were made to cover up improper care or to include something that was never done for or to the patient. Destruction or alteration of a medical record by an unauthorized person is known as *spoliation*.[6] To prevent the appearance of spoliation, health care providers should follow two simple rules:

1. When correcting an error, make a single line through the incorrect statement, initial and date the entry, and make the correct entry in the record. Attempting to obliterate the erroneous entry by whiting it out or scratching through the entry in such a way that a person cannot determine what was originally written sends up a red flag to someone looking for negligent or inappropriate care.

2. Entries in a medical record should be made on every line. Skip-

ping lines leaves room for tampering with records, a practice not in the best interest of patient or provider.

Failure to place the appropriate time of a procedure or treatment can be problematic if additional tests or treatments are ordered and the timing of such procedures is contingent on knowing when the other exam was performed. If the facility has not adopted military time (0100 to 2400), it is imperative that the appropriate designation of A.M. or P.M. be placed after the time noted in the chart. Including the starting and ending time of a procedure will allow the facility to track patient flow and length of studies, as well as determine a series of events if an incident arises with a patient.

Follow-up orders must always be included in a chart. Patient recovery and safety may be contingent on certain activities or behaviors (for instance, lie flat for eight hours, do not bend the leg for four hours). Failure to include follow-up instructions in a patient chart or in materials the patient takes along as an outpatient may result in liability for negligence if it can be determined that the failure to include such instruction caused the patient to be injured.

## Improper Charting

It is important to document all information that will assist in a patient's treatment. However, there are certain things that should *not* be included in the patient's medical record. Examples of inappropriate charting information include reference to or inclusion of an incident report, derogatory comments about the patient or a physician, opinion as to care rendered a patient, and opinion as to the correctness of an order given by a physician.

### Incident Reporting

Reference to or indication that an incident report was written concerning a patient or the incident report itself should never be included in a patient's medical record. However, information concerning an incident is very important to the facility. Therefore, the completed documentation should be sent to the appropriate hospital personnel. The risk manager, safety director, or designated responsible party will use the information for investigative and tracking purposes.

Some states require that incident reports pertaining to a patient be included in the patient record. If this is the case, the report should be drafted according to the requirements of documentation and included in the record.

Included in the record or not, incident reports should be factual accounts of perceived or actual incidents. Blame or finger pointing should not be part of the report. Only information that is known or was witnessed by the person completing the form should be incorporated into the form. Hearsay is not acceptable when writing factual accounts.

## *Derogatory Comments*

A medical record should be a positive accounting of the patient's diagnosis, treatment, and progress. Derogatory comments concerning the patient, the physician, another provider, or the facility have no place in the record. Liability may arise from any number of sources against a person who made an inappropriate comment in a patient's chart. For example, a technologist writes in a patient's chart that Doctor X incorrectly ordered a procedure because he is incompetent and was under the influence of drugs when he wrote the order. Other health care providers read this notation and begin to spread gossip concerning the physician throughout the hospital. In light of this gossip, other doctors refuse to refer patients to Dr. X because he's an "addict." Dr. X's patient load falls off, and he is subject to ridicule among physicians and in the health care community at large. Dr. X probably has an actionable claim against the technologist for defamation based on the fact that he has been subjected to ridicule in the community and that he has lost business because of the derogatory comment written in the chart.

Channels of communication are available for a technologist or therapist who believes that an inappropriate order has been written in a chart. Questioning the ordering physician in a professional and rational manner is the first step in rectifying the perceived error. If the physician does not give a reasonable explanation for the order or does not change the order after a healthy, intelligent discussion, then the technologist or therapist should go to a supervisor or other administrative personnel for clarification. Although technologists or therapists do not, except in special circumstances, have the right to order procedures, they do have a professional responsibility to question an order that does not appear to follow a prescribed protocol or match a history given by the patient. They do not, however, have the right to include derogatory comments concerning a physician or patient in a chart.

## OWNERSHIP OF RECORDS

There are several theories as to who owns a patient's medical record. Historically, it was recognized that the records belonged to the caregiver and that the patient had no right to even review the information contained in the record. This philosophy arose from the position that the physician was responsible for the care and well-being of the patient and that the patient should without question follow his or her orders.

As the relationship between physicians and patients changed and the ethical concept of personal autonomy became an important aspect of health care delivery, the ownership of or right to information from medical records also changed. The current widely accepted philosophy about medical records is that the caregiver or facility owns the records, but the patient has the right to the information included in the record except where prohibited by law or by the patient's medical condition.

The laws on ownership are as varied as the states themselves. Some states require that the records be released to patients upon request; others state that the patient must show cause, the records must be subpoenaed by the state, or there must be evidence that malpractice or negligence has occurred. A minority of states allow a summary of the patient's record to be released instead of the entire record.[7] Federal health care facilities are generally required to release a copy of the patient's medical record upon request.[8]

## Release of Records and Diagnostic Images

Most states consider radiographs and other images part of the medical record. Requirements for release of medical records vary from state to state. For example, in Georgia, upon written request from the patient, the provider having custody and control of the record shall furnish a complete and current copy to the patient, to any other provider designated by the patient, or to any person designated by the patient.[9] The reasonable cost of copying the records shall be covered by the person requesting the records.[10]

New statutory language in Kentucky requires that providers supply the first copy of the record to the patient at no charge.[11] It is not clear whether the cost of copying radiographs is included in this new law. Since copying radiographs can be a financial burden on a facility, if health care providers cannot charge a reasonable fee for copying radiographs, the consumer will probably pay for this cost in increased fees for other services. The majority of states allow health care providers to charge a reasonable fee for copying records; some even dictate the amount which may be charged. The cost of paper or copying film, as well as a portion of the cost of labor, usually may be passed on to the consumer in those jurisdictions where charging is neither prohibited nor dictated by statute or regulation.

Although records must be released, the originals or copies of the documents do not need to be handed over immediately upon request. A reasonable period between the request for and delivery of records is recognized by most state laws. Although the requirements of release vary from state to state, a few simple guidelines will help providers determine the best method for releasing records without disrupting the department or running afoul of state statutes or regulations.

# Record Release System

Facilities may adopt the following guidelines to set up a system that will work in the specific health care setting.

1. Develop a facilitywide policy for release of records.
2. Post the current legal requirements for release of records in the front office, file room, or other area where records are maintained.
3. Require the patient or legal representative to sign a release before any diagnostic images are removed from the department.
4. Do *not* release originals unless required by law or accrediting agencies. If the original must be released, make copies to be retained by the facility.
5. Establish reasonable fees for copying radiographs and written records.
6. Keep a log of any released records, including the patient's name; where films were released, such as physician's office, lawyer, or patient; date of release; number and type of films released; and date of return if applicable.
7. Educate all facility employees on the importance of maintaining all patient records, including diagnostic images.

Every facility, even a small physician's office, must develop a policy for film release. After all, the diagnostic images are the records that can verify that a procedure was completed in the facility and can justify a diagnostic interpretation if questioned in a court of law or other arena.

Lost or unreturned films can pose serious problems to a facility. If a legal claim is made against a facility or a provider, the radiographs may be the evidence needed to demonstrate that medical negligence or malpractice did or did not occur. When films are lost, or released and not returned, the courts may make one of three assumptions: (1) that the films were never taken; (2) that malpractice occurred (prima facie), the presumption being that the films are not available for a reason (to cover up malpractice); or (3) that malpractice occurred, with the burden of proof shifting to the defendant to show that negligence did not occur.

Any of these assumptions places a great burden on the defendant. Therefore, it is imperative that the facility's records policy include a very well thought-out and strict film release policy, preferably with a statement that original records *never* be released.

# Maintenance of Diagnostic Imaging Records

Just as there are statutes governing when and how records are to be released, there are also laws to determine how and for what period records should be maintained. Every state has requirements concerning how and for what period records are to be stored by a facility. Common elements of record maintenance are: (1) films must be maintained in a secure area with limited public access; (2) copies of the written interpretation should be maintained with the films as well as with the patient's medical record; (3) voluminous records may be stored in another area or placed, if economically feasible, on microfilm and stored in a secure area.

The length of time radiographs are to be maintained is usually determined by state law. The average period for keeping the images is five years for adults. In the case of minors, films generally need to be maintained until the minor reaches majority, usually eighteen, plus a statutory period ranging from one to seven years.[12]

Films should also be maintained if the facility has any indication that litigation may arise either from the care given, the occurrence of an incident, or because of statements made by or concerning a patient. All records gathered under these circumstances should be kept in a locked area, so that there is no possibility that records including radiographs and other images will be tampered with or removed from the facility.

## CONCLUSION

Documentation and maintenance of records, including diagnostic images, is a very important aspect of health care delivery. The patient, caregiver, and facility can all be protected if the facility maintains accurate and complete records. It is imperative that all facilities, regardless of size or scope of services, establish a policy concerning medical records, including content, storage, security, and release. Every employee in the facility must understand the importance of maintaining the quality and integrity of the record.

## N O T E S

1. Medical Records Services, *Accreditation Manual for Hospitals* (Oakbrook Terrace, Ill.: Joint Commission on Accreditation of Health Care Organizations, 1992).
2. Michael W. Drafke, *Trauma and Mobile Radiography* (Philadelphia: F. A. Davis, 1990), 122.
3. "Radiologic Technologists shall not diagnose, but in recognition of their responsibility to the patient, they shall provide the physician with all information they have relative diagnosis to patient management." American Society of Radiologic Technologists, *Code of Ethics for Radiologic Technologists*, Principle Seven.
4. Philip W. Ballinger, *Merrill's Atlas of Radiographic Positions and Radiologic Procedures* (St. Louis: Mosby-Yearbook, 1991).
5. Ibid.
6. "**Spoliation** . . . . 3. (Law) The destruction or alteration of a document by an authorized person." *Webster's New World Dictionary*, 2nd coll. ed. (Springfield, MA: 1982). "Spoliation . . . The destruction of evidence. It constitutes an obstruction of justice. The destruction, or the significant alteration of a document or instrument." *Black's Law Dictionary*, 5th ed. (St. Paul: West, 1979).
7. Public Citizen's Health Research Group, Washington, D.C.

8. Army Regulation 40-66, Medical Record Administration, July 20, 1992.
   §1-5 Record Ownership
   a. Army medical records are the property of the government . . .
   b. Army records will remain in the custody of the military . . . Upon request, the patient may be provided with a copy of his or her record but not the original record.
9. Georgia Code Annotated, §31-33-2, a–b.
10. Georgia Code Annotated, §33-33-3.
11. Kentucky Revised Statutes.
12. Mississippi Code 1972 Annotated 41-9-69 Retention of Records:
   Records must be maintained:
   Adults—Seven years if discharged at death
       Ten years if of sound mind
   Minors—Majority plus seven years not to exceed 28 years

# BIBLIOGRAPHY

*Comprehensive Accreditation Manual for Hospitals.* Oakbrook Terrace, Ill.: Joint Commission on Accreditation of Health Care Organizations, 1995.

Drafke, Michael W. *Trauma and Mobile Radiography.* Philadelphia: F. A. Davis, 1990.

Pozgar, George D. *Legal Aspects of Health Care Administration.* Rockville, Md.: Aspen Publications, 1993.

Scott, Ronald W. *Legal Aspects of Documenting Patient Care.* Rockville, Md.: Aspen Publications, 1994.

Torres, Lillian S. *Basic Medical Techniques and Patient Care for Radiologic Technologists.* 4th ed. Philadelphia: Lippincott, 1993.

C H A P T E R

# 7

# Standard of Care, Patient Rights, and Informed Consent

Ann M. Obergfell

$\mathbf{T}$o understand the role of diagnostic imaging and therapeutic personnel in a variety of health care settings, it is necessary to review the standard of care for the radiologic sciences, fundamental patient rights, and
the associated informed consent. Each of these concepts helps define the
way health care ought to be delivered, and each should be analyzed independently to better understand how the three are related.

## STANDARD OF CARE

In medical negligence and malpractice cases, the standard of care is
applied to measure the competence of the professional. The traditionally
recognized standard of care required that the medical professional practice his or her profession with the average degree of skill, care, and diligence exercised by members of the same profession practicing in the same
or similar locality in light of the present state of medical and surgical
practice.[1] As medicine has advanced through specialization, and as
quicker and more accurate communication methods have evolved, the
law has adapted and changed in most courts to disregard the previously
described geographical considerations and to set the standard as that of
a reasonable specialist practicing in the same field.[2] Therefore, individuals
practicing in the radiologic sciences must maintain the same level of com-

petence as a reasonable radiologic science practitioner in the same area of specialty.

When applying this principle to diagnostic imaging and therapeutic specialists, the liability issues increase as radiographers, nuclear medicine technologists, radiation therapists, and sonographers, depending on the limitations of state statutes and regulations, cross over specialization lines and practice in fields in which they have limited education and experience. Radiographers perform nuclear and sonographic studies as well as therapeutic procedures; nuclear technologists perform sonographic procedures; and sonographers swing back and forth across lines of specialization. Many members of these groups hold credentials in more than one field and are thereby qualified to cross lines and meet the standard of the specialty in which they practice, but a large percentage are trained on the job with limited direction and supervision.

Individuals with limited education and experience, who practice as those with the appropriate education and experience, will be expected to perform in the same manner as qualified personnel. A radiographer performing nuclear studies will be held to the standard of a nuclear medicine technologist and not to that of a radiographer practicing nuclear medicine. Health care facilities that require employees to perform procedures beyond the employee's educational expertise will be ultimately liable for the employee, but the employee will remain personally liable for all professional activity.

## Educational Standard

The educational requirements that determine the standard are generally those recognized by the profession as appropriate for the field. In radiography, nuclear medicine, radiation therapy, and sonography, educational essentials have been developed that define what an accredited program must do to educate students.[3] Curriculum guides for the radiologic sciences also define specific areas of study and propose associated content for each area.[4] The educational essentials and the curriculum guides are periodically reviewed and revised to meet the changing needs of the profession.

These educational requirements will be reviewed to determine whether a person practicing in a certain field has the requisite education. Attorneys may also review the continuing education requirements and the information available in scholarly journals and other periodicals to determine the standard of practice for a certain professional field.

The educational standard should be met by all personnel practicing in the radiologic sciences and associated fields. Technologists and therapists should obtain and maintain certification or registration in their area of expertise. Likewise it is imperative that technologists, therapists, and sonographers understand the standard for the field in which they practice and maintain currency in the field by attending continuing education programs and reading published articles and professional materials.

## Professional Standard

The standard reviewed to determine the appropriate professional practice is generally that recognized by the discipline's national professional organization. The standard may be in the form of a scope of practice or a series of guidelines set forth to determine what these health care specialists should and should not do under certain circumstances.[5] Individuals practicing in these fields should be familiar with these professional requirements and should upgrade their knowledge of professional practice as the standards change and develop.

Professionals who become stagnant or refuse to change the way they practice may be personally liable if they fail to meet the recommended standards of the profession. Many believe that, if they learned it in school, it is the right thing to do but should be reminded that just because it was learned in school does not mean it is still appropriate practice ten or twenty years later. People expect their physician to be current in his practice, and the same would be expected of diagnostic imaging and therapeutic specialists.

The radiologic sciences are changing rapidly, and it is incumbent on those who practice in these specialized fields to remain current. Inadequate time and money are generally not considered good reasons for being unprepared for changes in a field. Hospitals should maintain library facilities containing professional journals from many health care disciplines and offer in-service programs for employees. Public libraries carry the same or similar periodicals, and educational programs are required to maintain library resources which are usually available to members of the profession.

The standard of care recognized by the law should be the same level of care that a patient can expect and receive when entering a health care facility for professional service. Many patients' rights are based on the recognized standard of care and should be reviewed in this context.

## PATIENT RIGHTS

The relationship between health care professionals and patients has been analyzed from both the patient's and the professional's perspective. The two viewpoints are often in conflict, and it is important to review each perspective to find a method for peaceful and beneficial coexistence. The fundamental difference is that the long-recognized professional obligation to do what is necessary to help the patient may run counter to the patient's right to decide what will happen to his or her own body. For example, a patient enters the hospital with a pneumothorax, and the doctor recommends placement of a chest tube to relieve the condition, but the patient refuses the treatment. In this case, the treatment that is necessary to help the patient is being refused by the patient. While the patient's rights are paramount, it is easy to see how the principles may come into conflict.

The professional's responsibilities are generally laid out in guidelines such as the Code of Ethics for Radiologic Technologists, drafted by the American Society of Radiologic Technologists and adopted by the American Registry of Radiologic Technologists.[6] The patient's rights, at least in the hospital setting, are enumerated in the American Hospital Association's Patient Bill of Rights.[7]

## Professional Responsibility

Professionals are looked to as responsible individuals in several areas. The first is in the area of ethical principles and moral rules. Health care professionals—in particular, radiologic technologists—have an ethical code requiring that the technologist advance the principal objective of the profession to provide services to humanity with full respect for the dignity of mankind.[8] This lofty moral ideal lays a framework for the radiologic technologist and the day-to-day practice of diagnostic imaging. Another ethical requirement asserts the responsibility of the technologist to assess situations; exercise care, discretion, and judgment; assume responsibility for professional decisions; and act in the patient's best interests.[9] These and other ethical responsibilities are the foundation for practice in the radiologic sciences.

States may adopt guidelines for professional practice, either through statutes or by authorizing other state agencies to draft regulations to define appropriate practice. Such statutes or regulations may dictate who may practice in the profession, how they practice, how they must interact with patients, and what they must do to maintain their license or certificate.

The underlying ethical principle that dictates the professional responsibility of technologists is respect for patient autonomy. If technologists were to abide by this principle, there would be no conflict between professional responsibility and patient rights. Since most ethical codes and administrative regulations emphasize the duties of the professional rather than the rights of the patient, it is important to review the patient's rights as delineated by the American Hospital Association's Patient Bill of Rights.

## Patient's Rights

In the 1970s, patient rights became a greater concern of the health care community. To enhance and protect patient rights, the American Hospital Association first adopted its bill of rights in 1973. The document, revised and updated in October 1992, lists basic rights that ought to be enjoyed by hospital patients.[10]

The bill of rights was drafted and updated in an attempt to clarify basic fundamental rights of the patient. Although many of these rights are well established, patients often do not know what to ask or whom to ask if they have questions about their care, their health care charges, or their caregivers' obligations in the health care setting.

The document adopted by the American Hospital Association incorporates many patient rights, including the right to have an advance directive concerning treatment or to designate a surrogate decision maker.[11] Many states have living will or advanced directive statutes which permit citizens to make decisions, before they are ill or incapacitated, concerning the types of care they would elect or decline for themselves if able. Other statutes allow people to select a person, called a *health care surrogate*, to make decisions for them in the event they are unable to make their own decisions. The statutes vary from state to state, and some may limit the power to make decisions, as in the case of pregnancy.[12]

Another important patient right is the right to every consideration of privacy[13] and the right to expect that all communication and records pertaining to care will be treated as confidential by the hospital—except in special circumstances, such as suspected abuse or public health hazards, as is permitted or required by law.[14]

A regular concern of patients is whether there will be access to receive medical care. Under the bill of rights, the patient has the right to expect that the hospital, within its capacity and policies, will make reasonable response to a patient's request for appropriate and medically indicated care and services.[15] The patient may also review medical records and may request explanation of anything that is not clear or not understood, as long as this is permitted by law.[16] Access to records may be denied if, in the best professional judgment of the patient's physician, review of the records may cause emotional or psychological harm to the patient.

## INFORMED CONSENT

The most interesting and important, yet often ignored, fundamental patient right is the principle of personal autonomy, or the basic right to decide what will be done to one's own body. This fundamental human right was articulated in an early twentieth-century legal case which stated that every person of adult years and sound mind has the right to determine what happens to his body and that a physician who performs an operation without the patient's consent may be guilty of assault.[17] Selection of a health care alternative may be one of the most difficult decisions that a person will have to make during his or her lifetime. The patient must be offered enough information so that a rational and intelligent decision can be made and informed consent given.

The information necessary to make informed decisions includes the benefits and risks of the procedure, alternative procedures and treatments which may give the same or similar results, and the risks of electing no treatment.

The process for obtaining consent need not be complicated but should be designed in such a way that it meets the requirements of consent and centers on the concerns of the patient.

## Obtaining Consent

Physicians are the only health care professionals recognized under the law to obtain consent from a patient. Since the general public has little or no knowledge of medicine or medical practice, the average patient must rely on a physician to offer appropriate information about the nature of the care proposed. The physician has a duty to disclose all information which may affect the decision-making process.

Historically, courts utilized the standard of the medical community or measured the disclosure by "good medical practice," generally defined as that which a reasonable physician would have disclosed under the same or similar circumstances. These theories often utilized by the courts were found to be in conflict with the fundamental right of self-determination, since they removed the basic needs of the patient from the equation.

More recent cases have shifted the measure from that of the medical community to that of the patient's need to make the decision. In fact, the leading case found that it is the prerogative of the patient, not the physician, to determine personally the direction in which his or her interests lie.[18] The standard is objective but does not require that the physician "read the patient's mind" to determine what information is needed to make an intelligent and informed decision. The physician is required to use medical knowledge and experience to determine what information a reasonable person would need to know in order to make an informed and educated decision. In most cases, the nature of the relationship with the patient places the physician in the best position to know the patient's need for information and emotional stability.

The amount of information that needs to be given will vary from patient to patient but generally requires information about the benefits of the procedure; the accompanying risks, including the possibility of death or paralysis, no matter how minuscule the risk; reasonable procedure alternatives which the patient may elect; and the risks of electing no treatment. The patient needs this information to make a decision, and because of the disparity between the knowledge of the physician and the knowledge of the patient, it is incumbent upon the physician to offer whatever information is necessary and available.[19]

Hospitals and clinics should not rely on the ordering physician to obtain consent. While most physicians are familiar enough with a procedure to understand its diagnostic value, many physicians have little if any understanding of the procedure and its associated risks. While the physician may understand that a CT scan may require the use of a contrast media, he or she may not be familiar with side effects and contraindications.

Assuming that a patient has been given the appropriate information by the ordering physician may place a health care facility at peril of failing in its duty to offer the appropriate information to a patient so that consent may be obtained. A department's practice of asking certain questions concerning previous studies, adverse reactions, and allergies leads a reasonable person to believe that there is a possibility of complications from the administration of contrast media. The department's failure to communicate with the patient may lead a patient to believe there are no associated hazards or risks.[20]

Although the consent process seems straightforward and relies heavily on the physician's assessment of the needs of the patient, there are two exceptions to the requirements of informed consent. The first is in the case of an emergency, when the patient is unconscious or otherwise unable to give consent and it would be medically contraindicated and would be detrimental to the patient's well-being not to begin a diagnostic and treatment plan. The second exception is in the case when a patient is not able to process the information or, upon disclosure, may become so emotionally distraught that a rational decision cannot be reached, impeding rational treatment. The second exception requires that a physician have reason to believe that, upon disclosure, the person will become emotionally distraught—not just that the patient might refuse a recommended diagnostic or treatment plan.

## Consent Process

The physician who obtains the patient's consent must consult with the patient about the recommended procedure. The procedure should be explained in terms or language that the patient understands. If the patient's native tongue is different from the physician's, an interpreter (a family member or patient advocate) should be used. Difficult medical terminology should be kept to a minimum but, if used, should be explained to the patient's satisfaction.

The physician should consult with the patient on the risks and benefits associated with the procedure or treatment plan, alternatives to the plan, and any risks associated with not having the procedure or treatment. The patient should be given ample opportunity to read the consent form, which has been explained, and ask questions concerning the proposed plan. The presentation should be factual and designed to inform the patient, not to frighten or to coerce.

## Consent Form

Clinics, offices, and departments should utilize consent forms designed to inform the patient of the procedure and to document consent. The form should be developed with input from the physician, personnel assisting or performing the procedure, risk managers, and legal counsel.

The form must conform to the requirements of the hospital and the state. States will vary on the requirements for consent, and it is imperative that the necessary elements required by law be included in the process and the form. The facility may elect to use a single standard form, but in doing so must comply with the requirements of specific information concerning procedures and associated risks (see Figure 7–1). Separate forms for each procedure requiring consent may also be adopted; again, they must conform to the requirements in form and content.

The form should include the patient's name, the procedure name, a brief description of the procedure using lay terminology, who will be performing the procedure, the benefits and risks of the procedure, and any reasonable alternative. Signature lines should be placed at the bottom of the form and should include a line for the person performing the consult, one for the patient or a legally recognized representative, and at least one line for a witness who will not participate in the procedure or treatment.

The time frame for obtaining consent will vary from state to state and by procedure or treatment. Some states require a 24- to 48-hour waiting period between consent and procedure. Others require that, after 24 hours, the patient should be consulted again. The time required may be contingent on the nature of the procedure and the specific circumstances. Cardiovascular studies and therapeutic treatments, for example, may require a longer lead time than an IVP. Emergency procedures may not allow for the same time as some elective or nonemergency studies or treatments.

The panel or committee that reviews departmental policy should determine the appropriate time frames for consent and should incorporate them in the department's policies.

---

### CONSENT TO PERFORM MYELOGRAM

**Note:** Cross out any paragraph that does not apply or for which there is no consent.

Name _____

Medical Record # _____

I, _____, hereby authorize
Dr. _____ to perform the following
procedure _____.

I have been informed that, during this procedure, a needle will be placed in the spine and a small amount of spinal fluid will be removed. Contrast media will be injected into the spinal column, and a series of radiographs will be taken.

The possibilities of complications from needle insertion include an accumulation of blood in the tissue at the site of insertion (hematoma).

The injection of contrast media may also have rare adverse reactions, ranging from hives to shortness of breath to temporary or permanent paralysis. In a very rare case, death may occur.

The benefits of the procedure as well as alternative procedures that could be used have been clearly explained to me, and I acknowledge that no guarantee or assurance has been made as to the results that may be obtained.

If the use of anesthesia is necessary, I authorize Dr. _____ to administer those medications he deems necessary, and I have been informed of the risks, benefits, and alternatives for the administration of the anesthetic agents.

*I certify that I have read and fully understand the above consent to perform the myelographic procedure, that the explanations referred to were made, and that all questions were answered to my satisfaction. All blanks and statements requiring the insertion of information were filled in, and the inapplicable paragraphs, if any, were crossed out before I signed.*

Date _____

_____
Signature of Patient/Legal
Guardian

Time _____

When patient is a minor or incompetent to give consent, the authorized legal guardian must sign.

_____    _____    _____    _____
Witness            Date       Witness            Date

---

■ FIGURE 7–1    **CONSENT TO PERFORM MYELOGRAM**

## Policy and Procedure on Consent

Facilities performing diagnostic studies and therapeutic treatments that require signed consent should develop appropriate policies and procedures for how consent will be obtained. The policy should meet the required elements outlined previously and should include any procedural requirements mandated by state or federal statute or regulation.

The policy should be included in the facility's procedure manual and must be reviewed regularly to ensure currency. All personnel involved with procedures or treatments requiring consent should be familiar with the policy and understand how it is to be implemented. To ensure that all personnel, including physicians, understand the policy, it is recommended that a committee be formed to determine which procedures require consent, develop the policy, and coordinate implementation. The committee should be composed of a variety of individuals, including a physician, a technologist or therapist, a patient advocate, a department administrator, and legal counsel or a risk manager.

Any procedure that requires an invasive technique should require some form of consent, as well as any procedure with associated risks such that disclosure may help the patient determine whether he or she will elect to have the procedure. Therapeutic procedures that have elements of risk and recovery also require consent. Upon determining those procedures that require consent, lists of benefits, risks, and alternatives as well as a description of the procedure should be incorporated into a consent form and the department policy.

The form should be reviewed by non-medically related persons to determine whether it meets the requirements for adequate information. The policy for obtaining consent, along with a copy of the form and an appropriate rationale, should be distributed to all interested parties, including referring physicians, nursing floors, specialty units, and anyone who might send patients to an imaging or therapy department.

The physician is responsible for consulting with the patient and obtaining consent. Technologists or therapists are responsible for ensuring that consent has been obtained and that the patient has consented to the procedure either orally or, if required by policy, in writing.

## Technologist and Therapist Role in the Consent Process

The department policy should require that those procedures determined to need written consent should not be performed until adequate consent has been obtained. It should require that the technologist or therapist review the patient's chart and ascertain whether the required written consent has been obtained. If upon review the technologist or therapist finds no signed consent form, he or she should not begin the procedure until the appropriate physician has been contacted or consent has been obtained from the patient.

Communicating with the patient will also help the technologist or therapist determine whether the appropriate information has been given to the patient. A review of the proposed procedure or treatment will allow the patient to ask additional questions about the procedure and will help the technologist ascertain what, if any, information the patient has been given. This process will give the patient another opportunity to receive information concerning care and how the health care team plans to proceed.

Patients may feel more comfortable with the technologist than with the physician and therefore may express concerns about the course of treatment which have previously been left unsaid. The technologist or therapist is also the person who will perform or actively participate in the procedure or treatment and therefore will be better able to answer the patient's questions.

Professional judgment may be necessary in cases of emergency or when medically contraindicated, but it is best not to perform a procedure without the patient's consent. Physicians, administrators, technologists, and therapists should all understand the consent policies and should make certain that the patient's fundamental right of self-determination is not denied.

## CONCLUSION

The standard of care, patient rights, and informed consent are important aspects of health care delivery. If diagnostic imaging and therapeutic science professionals understand the importance of these concepts and follow the accepted practice as defined by each theory, many of the problems that can arise in the health care setting will be avoided. Members of the professional community as well as members of the general public should be made aware of these concepts and how they work together to form a comprehensive, patient-focused plan centering on self-determination and personal autonomy.

## N O T E S

1. Gillette v. Tucker, 65 NE 865.
2. Bruni v. Tucker, 346 NE2d 673.
3. *Essentials and Guidelines for an Accredited Educational Program for the Radiographer.* Adopted by the Joint Review Committee on Education in Radiologic Technology, July 1, 1994.
4. American Society of Radiologic Technologists, *Curriculum Guide for Radiography Programs,* 1991.

5. American Society of Radiologic Technologists, *Scope of Practice for Radiologic Technologists,* 1990.
6. American Society of Radiologic Technologists, *Code of Ethics for Radiologic Technologists,* 1990.
7. American Hospital Association, *Patient's Bill of Rights,* 1992.
8. *Code of Ethics for Radiologic Technologists.*
9. Ibid.
10. *Patient's Bill of Rights.*
11. Ibid.
12. Kentucky Revised Statutes (KRS).
13. Ibid., Right 5.
14. Ibid., Right 6.
15. Ibid., Right 8.
16. Ibid., Right 7.
17. Schloendorf v. Society of New York Hospital, 105 NE 92 (1914).
18. Canterbury v. Spence, 464 F2d 772 (1972).
19. Truman v. Thomas, 611 P.2d 902 (1980).
20. Keel v. St. Elizabeth Medical Center, 842 SW2d 860 (1992).

C  H  A  P  T  E  R

# 8

# Labor Law: The Employer- Employee Relationship

Raymond L. Smith, Jr.

**D**iagnostic imaging managers and supervisors must be prepared to deal with, at times, extremely complex issues, in order not only to make the most appropriate decisions, but also to be certain that the decisions made and the actions implemented do not run afoul of federal or state labor and employment laws. Therefore, it is essential that managers and other supervisory personnel have at least a general understanding of the labor and employment laws that affect their decision-making processes. As a general rule, most state labor and employment laws mirror or substantially follow the existing federal labor and employment laws. Therefore, this chapter will focus on those federal labor laws that most frequently present themselves in a manager's or supervisor's day-to-day decision-making processes.

## LABOR LAWS AND UNIONS

The Labor-Management Relations Act (LMRA)[1] generally requires employers and unions to bargain in good faith over wages, hours, and other terms and conditions of employment. The LMRA specifically provides employees with the

> right to self-organization, to form, join, or assist, labor or-
> ganizations, to bargain collectively through representa-
> tives of their own choosing, and to engage in other con-
> certed activities for the purpose of collective bargaining
> or other mutual aid and protection, and shall also have
> the right to refrain from such activities.[2]

In adopting Section 7 of the LMRA, Congress provided employees with the right to select a single representative for the purposes of bargaining over terms and conditions of employment for a group of employees with a particular employer. Alternatively, the LMRA provides employees with the right to refrain from such self-organization activity. To support employees' rights to self-organize, the LMRA also strictly prohibits employers from interfering with employees in their endeavor to do so.

If an employer interferes with employees' Section 7 rights, it will have committed an unfair labor practice.[3] Congress specifically mandated that it is an unfair labor practice for an employer to

> 1. interfere with, restrain, or coerce employees in the ex-
>    ercise of the rights guaranteed in Section 7;
> 2. dominate or interfere with the formation or administra-
>    tion of any labor organization or contribute financial or
>    other support to it;
> 3. discriminate in regard to hire or tenure of employment
>    or any term or condition of employment to encourage
>    or discourage membership in any labor organization;
> 4. discharge or otherwise discriminate against an em-
>    ployee because he has filed charges or given testi-
>    mony under the Act;
> 5. refuse to bargain collectively with the representatives
>    of his employees.

Likewise, Congress recognized the potential for employee organizations (unions) to abuse the power they were being granted by Congress. The LMRA provides that it is an unfair labor practice for labor organizations or their agents to

> 1. restrain or coerce (A) employees in the exercise of
>    rights guaranteed in Section 7 [29 USCS 147]: . . . or
>    (B) an employer in the selection of his representatives
>    for the purposes of collective bargaining or the adjust-
>    ment of grievances;
> 2. cause or attempt to cause an employer to discriminate
>    against an employee . . . or to discriminate against an
>    employee with respect to whom membership in such
>    organization has been denied or terminated on some
>    ground other than his failure to tender the periodic
>    dues and the initiation fees uniformly required as a
>    condition of acquiring or retaining membership;
> 3. refuse to bargain collectively with an employer;

4. (i) engage in, or to induce or encourage any individual employed by any person engaged in commerce or in an industry affecting commerce to engage in, a strike or a refusal in the course of his employment to use, manufacture, process, transport or otherwise handle or work on any goods, articles, materials, or commodities or to perform any services; or (ii) to threaten, coerce, or restrain any person engaged in commerce or in an industry affecting commerce, where in either case an object thereof is—
(A) forcing or requiring any employer or self-employed person to join any labor or employer organization . . . ;
(B) forcing or requiring any person to cease using, selling, handling, transporting, or otherwise dealing in the products of any other producer, processor, manufacturer, or to cease doing business with any other person, or forcing or requiring any other employer to recognize or bargain with a labor organization as the representative of his employees unless such labor organization has been certified as the representative of such employees . . . ;
(C) forcing or requiring any employer to recognize or bargain with a particular labor organization as the representative of his employees if another labor organization has been certified as the representative of such employees . . . ;
(D) forcing or requiring any employer to assign particular labor organization or in a particular trade, craft, or class . . . ;
5. picket or cause to be picketed, or threaten to picket or cause to be picketed, any employer where an object thereof is forcing or requiring an employer to recognize or bargain with a labor organization as the representative of his employees, or forcing or requiring the employer to select such labor organization as their collective bargaining representative, unless such labor organization is currently certified as the representative of such employees: . . .[4]

As is apparent from the above-quoted sections of the LMRA, Congress placed very specific and stringent restrictions on both employers and labor organizations regarding how the two entities should relate to one another. From management's perspective, the most critical concern is avoiding any violation of the LMRA by refusing to bargain in good faith with a labor organization when one requests representation status.

The federal labor relations laws are many and varied. However, by understanding the basic rights of employees, employers, and labor organizations under the LMRA, management will at least be prepared to avoid the most common complaints, administrative actions, or litigation in the labor field: unfair labor practice claims. The most effective means to avoid unfair labor practice claims is to prevent unionization of the workplace. If employers adequately educate management personnel not only to follow the employer's policies but also to respect its employees, much can be done to avoid employees' desiring outside union representation. In the practice of medicine, it is well established that the preventive treatment of a medical condition is far better than ignoring the condition until it must be treated. Basically, if an individual fails to treat a condition until it becomes more critical, the individual has less chance to recover. Likewise, if an employer simply ignores the complaints of its employees, those complaints may escalate to the point of poor employee morale and a desire for outside union representation. Therefore, certain actions should be taken to assure fair and consistent treatment of employees and, by doing so, avoid the threat of unionization.

## MANAGEMENT COMMITMENT TO AVOIDING UNIONIZATION

The decision to remain union free must emanate from the chief executive officer (CEO). Long- and short-range plans for employee relations should be developed in the same manner and with the same emphasis as those given to a new marketing program. Subordinate managers must be proactive in the fulfillment of their responsibility to maintain a union-free work environment. All levels of management and supervision must understand the CEO's personal commitment to an effective employee relations program. Serious attention should be given to middle managers' and first-level supervisors' concerns and suggestions about employee relations and the handling of employment problems. It is also essential that first-level supervisors be given proper training and supervision to ensure that they are handling employee relations with tact and diplomacy; supervisors should be *firm, but fair.*

First-level managers and supervisors play a key role in preventing unionization. The supervisor is management's direct link with each employee. Often an employee's perception of his immediate supervisor is his or her perception of the entire organization. All of an organization's efforts to develop effective personnel policies and procedures may be for naught if the supervisor does not administer those policies fairly and consistently.

Supervisors are not employees under the LMRA and are excluded from voting on or for union membership in the typical bargaining unit. Therefore, clearly, supervisors and managers must be fully committed to their organization's nonunion policy and must be active participants in helping the organization remain nonunion.

## Conditions That Could Lead to Unionization

When management fails to recognize the importance of employee complaints, employee morale is usually negatively affected. The following factors are typical warning signs of management's failure to effectively deal with employees, which consequently may create a work setting wherein employees will ultimately seek union representation:

1. Lack of training or care in screening applicants.
2. Failure to remove misfits or troublemakers, preferably during probation.
3. Failure to recognize leadership talent among employees and use it in the company's best interests.
4. Overqualified or higher-paid people expected to do lower-qualified or lower-paid work.
5. Lack of continuing courtesy, respect, and fair consideration from managers, supervisors, payroll people, and others.
6. Failure to *listen to* and *understand* the employee *before* making decisions or responses.
7. Failure to pay wages comparable to the job market.
8. Failure to persuade employees that wage and benefit terms are reasonable, just, and proper.
9. Poor housekeeping with relatively shabby or unkempt employee facilities, lavatories, eating areas, parking, and so on.
10. Failure to give good employees a sense of security and a feeling that they have a job that others want.
11. Handing out nasty "surprises" in work schedules, time off, work assignments, pay cuts, or other changes.
12. Failure to truthfully communicate what employees need to know about the company and their jobs.
13. Promises that are not kept, or promises that are vague and uncertain.
14. Failure to persuade employees that any criticism or discipline is for *their* benefit, not solely for the company's benefit.
15. Having a "small" person for a boss: one who sets a bad example, is snobbish or has a little clique of favorites.
16. Self-sufficient administrative aides who go ahead with actions and decisions beyond their real expertise.
17. Having a work environment where employees do not feel free to discuss their complaints or problems with management.
18. Having weak supervisors who constantly pass the buck to top management.

If any or all of these conditions exist in the employment setting, it is likely that some or all employees in that setting would at least be interested in finding out more about union representation and, potentially, in obtaining such representation. In the event these conditions do exist, management should take the time to ascertain whether any union activity is already occurring in the workplace.

## Common Signs of Union Activity

To determine whether any type of union activity exists in the workplace, it is essential that managers and supervisors be aware of any changes in usual or normal employee behavior or attitudes. The following are some examples of employee behavior that could indicate union activity:

1. Employees meet and talk in out-of-the-way places.
2. The same employee is seen going to the washroom with several different workers during the day. He or she could be trying to sign them up.
3. Employees pass out material or union cards.
4. Employees arrive unusually early or leave late, and hang around or meet with other workers.
5. Certain employees are getting new or unusual amounts of attention.
6. Respected and popular employees suddenly become unpopular.
7. Employees from separate departments or different job levels begin meeting and talking together.
8. Nonunion people begin meeting and talking with known union members.
9. Employees start leaving the premises for lunch or are absent from customary social get-togethers.
10. Abnormal absenteeism.
11. New leaders arise among employees.
12. The nature and frequency of employee complaints change.
13. Complaints are made by a delegation, not by single employees.
14. Unusual employee questions about company policy and practices. This could mean a union attempt to document a case against you.
15. Employees who were previously relaxed or aimless are very busy or excited at break time.
16. The nature of rumors on the grapevine changes drastically, or the grapevine shuts down.
17. Flash rumors. An increase in rumors could mean employee insecurity or agitators trying to lower morale by raising doubts in employees' minds.

18. Strangers appear on company premises or in work areas.
19. Employees are being followed home from work. This is one way a union organizer can get home addresses for future house calls.
20. People start needling a single worker about the location of his workstation or the condition of his tools or equipment.
21. Down-to-earth employees develop social consciousness or become advocates for causes of other employees.
22. Good workers begin doing poor work.
23. Poor workers begin doing good work.
24. Employees hang around with fired employees.
25. Employees avoid being seen with managers or supervisors.

If management notices that any of the above activities or warning signs exist in their workplace, then certain prompt and immediate steps should be taken to attempt to diffuse the situation and avoid its escalation into a union recognition request or petition.

## Handling Union Activity

Any manager or supervisor who becomes aware of or even suspects that an employee is engaged in union activity should immediately report that fact to his or her supervisor, who in turn should immediately communicate such information to the hospital's or organization's legal department or outside counsel. It is vital that top management be made aware of any such activity as soon as possible. The rules change drastically once actual organizational activity has begun, and management must be in a position to react quickly. Furthermore, as noted above, there are a number of legal restraints imposed on employers, their managers, and supervisors during a union organizational campaign. To remember the rules, just think of the acronym TIPS. In other words, a manager or supervisor may not Threaten employees as a result of their union activity, may not Interrogate about union activities, may not Promise employees pay increases, promotions, or improved benefits on the condition that the employee refuse to join the union; and supervisors and managers may not Spy on or engage in Surveillance of employees attending union meetings or receiving handbills from union supporters.

A violation of these rules could result in an unfair labor practice charge being filed against the hospital or organization and, in certain circumstances, could cause the National Labor Relations Board (NLRB) to issue an order requiring the hospital to recognize and bargain with the union without ever having an election among the employees.

There is no absolute method of avoiding unionization. The more time and attention a hospital or organization pays to its employees, the less it has to fear from unions. The extent to which the hospital or organization is willing to invest the time and effort in remaining union free is a management decision.

The key in remaining union free is effective, ongoing communication with employees. It is important that management not assume that employees understand and appreciate what the hospital or company does for them. Management should establish itself as the vehicle for information for its employees. Employees should look to the employer and its supervisors for information. If employees do not feel free to communicate with management and management is not responsive (simply listening and responding need not mean that management gives in), then employees could become interested in unionization.

## Remaining Union Free

The statement "Unions are a substitute for poor management" is often a truism. The key to a successful preventative labor relations program is good management and good employee communication.

Most employees who cast their votes for union representation do not vote "for" the union, they vote "against" management. Generally, employees who support a campaign for unions do so out of resentment toward their managers or supervisors.

Supervisors must be aware that employees are often troubled by many small and seemingly insignificant job-related problems. These problems, however, can grow into major sore points if they are not given immediate and serious attention by someone on the management team. *Prompt attention by supervisors to employee complaints, questions, or problems is essential.* Even if the employee is eventually unhappy with the action taken by management, if the employee is convinced that an effort was made by somebody on behalf of management to consider the problem fairly and to promptly report back, that employee is better able to accept management's decision than when management simply refuses to even consider the problem or fails to follow through with the employee.

Employers can minimize the risk of unionization and other legal problems by:

1. Keeping employees well informed.
2. Treating each employee with dignity and respect, as an individual.
3. Knowing and understanding employee needs, problems, and motivations.
4. Resolving complaints, questions, and problems as promptly as possible.

5. Being a good listener, encouraging ideas and suggestions and following up.
6. Disciplining employees fairly by consistent and uniform enforcement of work rules.

Obviously, the best way to prevent unionization is to make it unnecessary in the first place. To the people who work for a manager, the manager is the company, and the way managers treat employees has a tremendous influence on their behavior and attitude toward the company and toward unionization. Of course, managers have to know what employees want before anything can be done to meet employees' needs. Surprisingly enough, *money isn't always most important to employees.* Managers can't motivate employees to perform better and can't meet their needs simply by paying attention to their hourly rate and giving them a wage increase once a year. *Management has to know what is really important to employees, not what they think should be most important.*

The most important and essential aspect of remaining union free is to properly train managers and supervisors on how to handle personnel decisions. To do this, hospitals and other organizations must familiarize management personnel with the organization's policies and procedures and antidiscrimination laws. In addition, it is essential that, in taking personnel actions, management document disciplinary problems and personnel actions. However, any documented reference to unionization, age, race, or gender in connection with an employment decision can provide a basis for a legal complaint.

In addition, it is imperative that policies and procedures be current. Over the last ten years, numerous court decisions have eroded the standard employment at-will policy of most states and employers. Generally, absent a contract of employment or a union collective bargaining agreement, most employees are employed at-will. The phrase "employed-at-will" basically means the employee or the employer may terminate the employment relationship at any time, for any reason not prohibited by law, such as because of race or gender. However, as stated, numerous judicial decisions have eroded the at-will policy and found that, at times, an employer's employee policies or handbook can be the basis for establishing a modification of the employment at-will relationship and an enforceable contract of employment.

Because of this erosion of the at-will policy, it is imperative that employee policies and handbooks be job related and not unfairly penalize employees. Policies should include a philosophy on unionization, equal employment opportunity and should be widely and regularly disseminated. Probably the most basic and important requirement of personnel policies is that they treat all employees uniformly and that they are applied by management consistently.

---

## ESTABLISHING EFFECTIVE EMPLOYEE APPRAISAL SYSTEMS

Ineffective performance appraisal systems can lead to unionization as well as to claims of discrimination and unjust discharge. A typical appraisal system should meet the following criteria, which will also make it easier to defend in court:

1. Management follows specific guidelines on how to complete appraisals.
2. The system is behavior oriented rather than trait oriented.
3. Job analysis forms the basis of the appraisal system.
4. Employees' performance is evaluated by more than one supervisor.
5. Appraisal is not totally subjective.
6. The employee is fully apprised of his or her appraisal.
7. The employee is given notice of performance deficiencies and an opportunity to improve.

In addition, management should designate someone, such as the human resources manager, to oversee discharge and disciplinary actions to assure adherence to organization policies. Courts usually look favorably on discharge procedures that require several levels of approval. The personnel director should always seek to obtain the employee's explanation of the events leading to the disciplinary action and, if dismissal is involved, an exit interview can be most enlightening on how to avoid problems that may exist, not with the employee, but with a lower-level manager or supervisor.

For example, there are occasions when certain departments experience higher turnover than others. Management must recognize these situations and determine whether the employee turnover is the result of poor working conditions, unpleasant job duties, low pay, or, more importantly, poor or discriminatory management practices. Many times employee turnover can be attributed to abusive management practices which lead not only to poor employee morale, but also to the need or desire for outside union representation. In this regard, certain other preventive measures should be evaluated and, if needed, implemented:

1. Give employees fair warning of their deficiencies. Failure to do so creates potential exposure in employment termination litigation.
2. Keep full and proper documentation of actions taken against an

employee and the basis for those actions, including any progressive discipline taken.

3. When communicating with the employee, be sure to give the true reason for the action to be taken even if it is unpleasant. However, don't say too much, only what is necessary to explain the reasons for termination.

4. The company may want to establish some internal grievance or dispute resolution procedure, which can help to ensure that an employee is treated fairly and can provide several levels of review for personnel decisions.

5. The employer may want to consider granting severance pay or other benefits, *which the employee is not otherwise entitled to receive,* in return for a full release of all claims. Such releases are usually binding if done in accordance with necessary legal requirements.

6. The employer should have a consistent termination process.

## CONCLUSION

The practicalities of the employment relationship dictate that management recognize fair and consistent treatment and application of employment policies as the primary means of avoiding unionization. In addition, as will be discussed in Chapter 9, management's failure to treat employees uniformly and fairly can give rise to employee discrimination suits based on myriad civil rights laws.

### NOTES

1. 29 U.S.C. 141 et seq.
2. 29 U.S.C. 157 (LMRA Section 7).
3. 29 U.S.C. 158.
4. 29 U.S.C. 158.

# 9

# Employment Discrimination Law

Raymond L. Smith, Jr.

**B**oth state and federal laws prohibit discrimination in terms and conditions of employment on the basis of race, sex, age, national origin, religion, or disabled status. These antidiscrimination laws are applicable to and directly affect all employment decisions including hiring, firing, promotions, transfers, job assignments, discipline, benefits, and generally all other terms and conditions of employment. Although the laws involved are too numerous to discuss in detail, a brief overview of civil rights legislation is invaluable to the effective management of employee relations.

**Title VII of the Civil Rights Act of 1964**[1]   Title VII, as it is generally referred to, is the most recognized and litigated civil rights law in America. Title VII protects employees from discharge or discipline because of race, color, sex, religion, or national origin and from any retaliation for the exercise of these protected rights.

**Civil Rights Act of 1866**[2]   Pursuant to this statute, nonwhite citizens have the right to contract, sue, participate in legal proceedings, and enjoy the full benefits of the law. Since employee and employer relationships have been deemed contractual in nature, this statute has been judicially determined to be applicable to employment practices that infringe on the aforementioned protected rights.

**Civil Rights Act of 1871**[3]   This civil rights law protects employees from discriminatory employment actions when such actions amount to a deprivation of any right established by federal law or the United States Constitution, provided that the employer is acting under the color of law;

that is, as an agent of federal or state government. The act covers primarily race and sex discrimination against public, state, or federal employees.

**Equal Pay Act of 1964**[4]   This law prohibits discrimination in compensation on the basis of sex where employees of the opposite sex perform equal work on jobs requiring equal skill, effort, and responsibility; and perform under similar working conditions.

**Age Discrimination in Employment Act of 1967**[5]   The Age Discrimination Act protects employees ages forty and above from discrimination in terms and conditions of employment, including discharge, on account of age. The law applies to public and private employers.

**Rehabilitation Act of 1973**[6]   This law protects employees from discrimination in terms and conditions of employment, including discharge, because of disabled status. The law applies to federal agencies, executive branch departments, and certain private employers performing federal contracts or subcontracts.

**The Americans with Disabilities Act of 1990**[7]   The Americans with Disabilities Act (ADA) protects employees from discrimination in terms and conditions of employment, including discharge, because of disabled status, a perception of disability, or a record of physical or mental impairment. The law applies to private employers, employment agencies, labor organizations, and joint labor-management committees. The U.S. government and its employees are specifically exempted from coverage under the act. The law requires employers to make reasonable accommodations for disabled employees to provide them with equal employment opportunities.

**The Family and Medical Leave Act of 1993**[8]   This law requires certain private employers to permit employees to take up to twelve weeks' unpaid leave from their employment during any twelve-month period for one or more of the following reasons: birth of a child and to provide care for that child; adoption of a child; care for one's spouse, child, or parent with a serious health condition; or a serious health condition of the employee that affects the employee's ability to perform the functions of the position held with the employer. The law also protects employees from any discrimination due to such leave and provides employees with the right to an equivalent position, pay, and other terms and conditions of employment upon their return from leave.

## EMPLOYMENT DISCRIMINATION

As may be apparent from the summary of laws discussed above, employment discrimination laws are quite encompassing. However, the general elements of most discrimination laws can be identified and, without addressing the peculiarities of each of these laws, can provide management with a good working understanding of how these laws are applied and, more importantly, how to avoid these types of employee complaints. Generally, discrimination claims are based on a claim of disparate treatment, disparate impact, and/or retaliation.

## Disparate Treatment

When an employee believes that he or she has been treated differently than other similarly employed individuals, that employee may make a disparate treatment claim. A disparate treatment claim is based on discriminatory practices directed at a particular employee. The employee may prove that the employer intended to discriminate against him or her by circumstantial evidence showing that the employee was treated differently than similarly situated persons with other racial, religious, or gender characteristics. Courts will also look for any deviations by the employer in the application of its practices or policies directed toward that employee.

## Disparate Impact

Unlawful discrimination can also be found based on the application of company policies or practices that are neutral on their face (applied equally to all employees) but affects minorities or other protected employees at a greater rate than nonprotected employees. If minorities or other protected groups are disproportionately affected, then the policy must be job related and justified by business necessity or a disparate impact claim may be asserted.

## Retaliation

Many of the employment laws addressed above prohibit employers from retaliating against employees for exercising their statutorily protected rights to complain about discriminatory conduct. For example, Title VII and the Age Discrimination Act prohibit employers from retaliating against employees in any way for filing an Equal Employment Opportunity charge with the Equal Employment Opportunity Commission (EEOC).[9]

## The Prima Facie Case

The pivotal case addressing Title VII claims is *McDonnell Douglas v. Green*,[10] wherein the United States Supreme Court laid down a four-part test for establishing a prima facie case of employment discrimination. The complainant in a Title VII case carries the initial burden of establishing a prima facie case, which generally requires proof that (1) the complainant belongs to a protected class; (2) he or she applied for and was qualified for a position which the employer was seeking to fill; (3) despite his or her qualifications, he or she was rejected; and (4) the position remained open and the employer continued to seek applicants from persons of the complainant's qualifications. The formula provided by *McDonnell Douglas* deals on its face only with refusal-to-hire cases. However, it has been held to apply, with appropriate modification, to discriminatory practices in other terms and conditions of employment.[11] Similar prima facie tests exist for the other employment discrimination laws addressed above. Establishing a prima facie case does not mean that the employee has established that he or she was discriminated against. However, it does provide the proper foundation for the employee to file a charge of discrimination with the appropriate enforcement agency.

Probably the most prolific area of employment litigation involves claims of sexual harassment in the workplace. Consequently, it is imperative that management clearly understand this area of the law and educate their supervisors on how to effectively deal with employee complaints of sexual harassment.

## Prohibition Against Sexual Harassment in the Workplace

Title VII's prohibition against sex discrimination in employment has been consistently interpreted to include sexual harassment on the job.[12] The EEOC's guidelines[13] define sexual harassment as follows:

> (a)  Harassment on the basis of sex is a violation of Sec. 703 of Title VII. Unwelcomed sexual advances, requests for sexual favors, and other verbal and physical conduct of a sexual nature constitute sexual harassment when (1) submission to such conduct is made either explicitly or implicitly a term or condition of an individual's employment, (2) submission to or rejection of such conduct by an individual is used as the basis for employment decisions affecting such individual, or (3) such conduct has the purpose or effect of unreasonably interfering with an individual's work performance or creating an intimidating, hostile, or offensive working environment.

Following the EEOC's guidelines, courts have generally recognized two types of sexual harassment: quid pro quo and hostile working environment.

## Quid Pro Quo

Quid pro quo sexual harassment occurs when submission to sexual conduct is implicitly or explicitly made a term or condition of an employee's initial or continued employment, or is used as the basis for any employment decision affecting the individual employee. Thus, unlawful sexual harassment occurs if an employee is denied a promotion or a wage increase, is demoted or loses an opportunity for advancement, or is laid off or terminated because the employee refused to submit to sexual advances. Quid pro quo harassment necessarily involves a supervisor or manager.[14]

## Hostile Work Environment

Courts have also found unlawful sexual harassment where the harassing conduct unreasonably interferes with the employee's work performance or creates an intimidating, hostile, or offensive work environment. The U.S. Supreme Court originally recognized environmental sexual harassment as violative of Title VII in the case of *Meritor Savings Bank v. Vinson*.[15] The Court has recently refined its holding in *Meritor* so that an employee need not prove that the hostile environment was so severe that it seriously affected the employee's psychological well-being. According to the Court, the working environment must only be one that a reasonable person would find hostile or abusive and that the victim subjectively perceives as abusive.[16] Environmental sexual harassment can be caused by either supervisors, coworkers, or customers.

In a hostile environment case, unlawful sexual harassment will be found even though it does not result in the loss of a tangible job benefit.[17] Where an employer creates or condones a substantially discriminatory work environment, regardless of whether the complaining employee lost any tangible job benefits as a result of the discrimination, it will be liable for the sexually hostile working environment.

Environmental sexual harassment cases usually involve conduct such as sexual suggestions, sexually derogatory remarks, sexually motivated physical conduct, and other sexually suggestive remarks or items.

Generally, the elements of a prima facie case of environmental sexual harassment are as follows:

1. The employee must be a member of a protected class.
2. The employee must have been subjected to unwelcome sexual harassment in the form of sexual advances, requests for sexual favors, or other verbal or physical conduct of a sexual nature.
3. The complained-of harassment must have been based on sex.
4. The charged sexual harassment must have had the effect of unreasonably interfering with the plaintiff's work performance and created an intimidating, hostile, or offensive working environment that seriously affected the psychological well-being of the plaintiff.
5. *Respondeat superior* employer liability exists.

In *Harris v. Forklift Systems,*[18] the United States Supreme Court held that the fourth factor set forth above must be modified to reflect that an employee need not establish that the hostile environment "seriously affected" the psychological well-being of that employee. Notwithstanding this modification, the prima facie case is otherwise applicable. The court also recognized that psychological well-being is a term, privilege, or condition of employment within the meaning of Title VII. Nevertheless, to state a claim of sexual harassment under Title VII, the activity must be sufficiently pervasive to alter the conditions of employment and create an abusive working environment.

Whether sexual harassment at the workplace is sufficiently hostile or abusive to establish liability for the offending conduct is a question to be determined in light of all the circumstances of the employment relationship. The mere presence of an employee who has engaged in particularly severe or pervasive sexual harassment can, in some cases, create a hostile working environment.[19]

In determining whether the alleged conduct constitutes sexual harassment, the EEOC will investigate the nature of the sexual advances and the context in which the alleged incidents occurred. The determination of the legality of a particular action will be made from the facts, on a case-by-case basis.[20]

## Protected Persons

Men as well as women are protected from sexual harassment in the workplace. For example, one court found that a female supervisor sexually harassed a male state employee when she demoted him after he ended their consensual sexual relationship.[21]

Further, it has been held that both male and female employees are protected from a homosexual supervisor's sexual advances.[22] Title VII's prohibitions of sexual harassment extend to homosexual as well as heterosexual conduct.

However, Title VII does not extend to harassment that arises from a person's sexual preference. For example, a male employee, who contended that he was forced to resign as a result of physical and mental harassment by male coworkers who disapproved of his live-in relationship with another man, did not establish a prima facie case of hostile-environment sexual harassment because the harassment was based on sexual preference, not on gender.[23]

Title VII's prohibitions against sexual harassment have also been found to extend to consensual relations gone sour. Courts have held that a male supervisor unlawfully retaliated against a female employee who had terminated their consensual sexual relationship.[24]

The EEOC's guidelines also provide that where employment opportunities or benefits are granted because of an individual's submission to the employer's sexual advances or requests for sexual favors, the employer may be held liable for sex discrimination against other persons who were qualified for but denied that employment opportunity or benefit due to their failure or refusal to provide sexual favors.[25]

## Unwelcome Conduct

For conduct to be actionable as proscribed sexual harassment under Title VII, such conduct must be unwanted and offensive. For example, one court held that a plaintiff was not offended by a sexually explicit cartoon given her by a supervisor, in light of the fact that the workplace environment was one in which sexual horseplay was consensual and the plaintiff freely participated in telling sexual jokes. Likewise, the fact that she kept the cartoon belied her assertion that it offended her.[26] In a similar case, it was determined that a personnel director's harassment was not unwelcomed by the plaintiff, even though he paid extremely close attention to her, since she never made any realistic effort to cut it off. She shared many of her personal problems with him and never made serious demands on him to stop paying such close attention to her. The court found the plaintiff was sending out mixed signals in that her requests were not delivered with any sense of emergency, sincerity, or force.[27]

Another court found that sexual innuendo and vulgarity were commonplace in a female quality control shop, were indulged in by employees of both genders, including the plaintiff, and thus were not sufficient for a Title VII sexual harassment action.[28]

## EMPLOYER'S LIABILITY

National and local media routinely report jury verdicts that award victims of sexual harassment hundreds of thousands of dollars. These extreme cases are clearly the exception to the norm. However, because of the inflammatory nature of the claims and the evidence presented in such cases, such as explicit pornography and sexual aids, employers risk substantial exposure if they fail to deal promptly and adequately with employees' complaints of sexual harassment. It is imperative that supervisors and other management personnel be well trained in how to deal with such complaints. As will be shown, failure to educate management personnel on how to avoid or deal with sexual harassment in the workplace could result in substantial liability to the employer.

## Sexual Harassment by Supervisors

Generally, the EEOC's guidelines hold an employer responsible for sexual harassment by its agents and supervisory employees, regardless of whether the specific acts complained of were authorized or even forbidden by the employer, and regardless of whether the employer knew or should have known of their occurrence.[29]

Most courts have likewise imposed strict liability on an employer for quid pro quo sexual harassment by a supervisor or manager.[30] The courts are divided, however, on the issue of whether an employer is strictly liable when the sole result of the supervisor's behavior is the creation of a hostile work environment.

Though the United States Supreme Court has provided guidance on the question of employer liability, it set no bright line rule for making a determination in a hostile environment case.[31] The Eleventh Circuit Federal Court of Appeals has ruled that an employer would not be liable unless it knew or should have known of the sexual harassment and failed to take prompt remedial action.[32]

While other courts have held an employer strictly liable regardless of the employer's knowledge, one court found an employer not liable for a sexually hostile environment created by a supervisor who allegedly sexually assaulted a former employee. In that case, the court determined there was no evidence that sexual harassment was within the scope of the supervisor's employment, and the employer promptly suspended and then discharged the supervisor after being informed of the assault. Since the supervisor neither purported to act on behalf of the employer nor used or threatened to use his authority over the employee in carrying out the assault, even though he took advantage of the opportunity presented by the workplace to commit the offensive act, the employer was held not liable.[33]

## Harassment by Coworkers

The EEOC guidelines also impose liability on an employer for acts of sexual harassment in the workplace by coworkers, where the employer (or its agents or supervisory employees) knew or should have known of the offensive conduct and failed to take immediate and appropriate corrective action.[34]

An employer acts unreasonably if it either unduly delays its remedial action or if the action that it does take, however promptly, is not reasonably likely to prevent misconduct from recurring.[35] It has been held that an employer is not liable for sexual harassment by coworkers when it quickly responded to the employee's complaints of harassment, held meetings with the complaining employee, and transferred the employee to a different shift.[36]

Judicial decisions generally limit an employer's liability to situations where the employer had actual or constructive notice of the harassing conduct by coworkers and failed to take appropriate action. An additional limitation on employer liability is the requirement that the alleged offensive conduct be severe and pervasive, as opposed to sporadic or isolated incidents of offensive conduct. In *Harris v. Forklift Systems*, the Supreme Court held that mere offensive utterances do not as a matter of law rise to the level of actionable harassment.[37]

## Employer's Responsibility for Prevention and Prompt Remedial Action

The EEOC guidelines encourage employers to take steps to prevent sexual harassment from occurring. Once an employer is on notice of potential sexual harassment, it must take prompt and adequate remedial action.[38]

### Prevention

The EEOC's guidelines mandate that employers take affirmative steps to prevent sexual harassment:

> **Prevention is the best tool for the elimination of sexual harassment. An employer should take all steps necessary to prevent sexual harassment from occurring, such as affirmatively raising the subject, expressing strong disapproval, developing appropriate sanctions, informing employees of their right to raise and how to raise the issue of harassment under Title VII, and developing methods to sensitize all concerned.**

Based on the EEOC's guidelines and judicial decisions, employers should consider taking the following steps in order to prevent sexual harassment in the workplace:

■ Specifically include sexual harassment as prohibited activity in the employer's written nondiscrimination policy.
■ Conduct training programs for supervisors and management to advise them of the law, their responsibility, and the consequences to the employer and the manager should sexual harassment occur.
■ Designate one individual, preferably a respected member of management, to receive complaints of sexual harassment. Employees should not be required to take their sexual harassment complaints to their supervisors because the harasser may be the supervisor. It is generally a good idea to designate an alternate in the event that the primary designee is the alleged harasser.
■ Establish a procedure for handling sexual harassment complaints which includes documentation and thorough investigation. Avoid making the procedure unduly complicated or burdensome and, once it is established, be sure that it is followed in each case.
■ Take each complaint seriously. Resist the temptation to treat complaints as frivolous. The embarrassment and stress involved in complaining of sexual harassment may affect the complainant's ability to articu-

late the problem. Advise the complainant that an immediate investigation will be conducted.

- When a complaint of sexual harassment is raised by an employee, be careful to avoid retaliatory actions or employment decisions that may *appear* retaliatory against the complainant.
- In conducting an investigation and determining what action should be taken, employers must attempt to be fair to both the complainant and the accused.
- If the investigation reveals that a supervisor or other employee is guilty of sexual harassment, appropriate action should be taken immediately, including disciplinary action against the harasser. Keep a written record of the discipline taken and let the victimized employee know what has been done to protect his or her rights and personal dignity.
- Be discreet in conducting the investigation and do not reveal the complaint or other information gathered during the investigation to anyone in the company who does not need to know.
- Because credibility of the complainant and the accused generally becomes an issue, the investigator should inquire as to whether there are witnesses to substantiate the employee's sexual harassment complaint. If there are no substantiating witnesses, the employer should look for other indices that would support either party's version of what happened. This may require the investigator to talk with people who are familiar with both parties' professional conduct.
- Establish written guidelines to be used in making employment decisions, especially promotion and compensation decisions, and make sure they are followed.
- Do not permit sexual jokes, teasing, and innuendo to become a routine part of the work environment.

## Prompt and Adequate Remedial Action

Even if an employer were to take all the preventive steps outlined above, sexual harassment may occur. If it does, the employer's focus then must shift to remedying the offensive conduct and avoiding liability for the offender's actions. To avoid liability under Title VII, an employer on notice of sexual harassment must do more than indicate the existence of an official policy against such harassment. The employer must show that it took prompt and adequate remedial action.

The Ninth Circuit Federal Court of Appeals has set a standard for determining the effectiveness of an employer's attempt to stop purported sexual harassment. The court noted that the reasonableness of the employer's remedy for coworkers' sexual harassment will depend on its ability to stop the harassment.[39]

In another case, a court held that an employer's prompt investigation of the employee's allegations, along with prompt remedial measures which brought the incidents to a stop, supported a finding that the employer was not liable for the supervisor's creation of the hostile environment. The employer's remedial actions consisted of advising the supervisor that any conduct of the type alleged was intolerable to the company. The employer also required the supervisor to discuss the matter with the offended employee. The actions taken by the employer brought the improper conduct to a stop.[40]

What is appropriate action will depend on the circumstances. One court held that a bank took appropriate action in response to a complaint of sexual harassment by conducting a full investigation immediately after the complaint was received and reprimanding the supervisors involved by placing them on suspension and warning them that any further harassment would result in their discharge. The court specifically noted that Title VII did not require the bank to fire the wrongdoers.[41]

The discharge of sexual harassers has, however, been upheld in a number of cases. One court upheld the termination of a railway superintendent, who claimed he was wrongfully terminated because of his age, where the evidence established that he was terminated by the employer for engaging in sexual harassment of a female employee.[42]

Employers need to be cognizant of the fact that when taking steps to eliminate sexual harassment or to accommodate an offended employee, the action taken should not adversely affect the complaining employee. For example, transferring an offended employee to another available position, which is less desirable than the position previously held by the employee, could result in the employee claiming retaliation for complaining about the offender's conduct.

By this point, it should be uncomfortably apparent that decisions made by managers and supervisors can and do have the potential to substantially affect the operations of the employer, not to mention subject the employer to civil liability for its actions. However, employers have the potential for additional liability above and beyond that provided in the numerous labor and employment laws already discussed. Specifically, a typical employment discrimination complaint will also include any number of common law, nonstatutory claims, which generally have no limitations on the damages or relief available from a court or jury.

## OTHER LEGAL ISSUES

Generally, remedies under most antidiscrimination statutes are limited to reinstatement, back pay, attorneys' fees, and recovery of costs. Consequently, complaining employees frequently append common law tort claims to their statutory causes of action in order to request awards for compensatory, consequential, and punitive damages. The most typical common law claims appended to Title VII actions are discussed in the sections that follow.

## Assault and Battery

Usually, if physical touching is alleged in a sexual harassment case, the plaintiff will append a common law claim of *assault and battery*. Reference to state law is required to determine what a plaintiff must allege regarding the elements of an assault and battery claim; for example, whether physical contact is required and the degree of that contact.

## Intentional Infliction of Emotional Distress

Traditionally, a claim for *intentional infliction of emotional distress* has required proof of physical injury. However, many courts have held that, in the sexual harassment context, plaintiffs do not need to show the element of physical injury.

In one case, a manager's conduct included threats and attempts to use his authority to force plaintiff to acquiesce to his sexual advances. The court found that when the plaintiff rejected the sexual advances, the plant manager's mistreatment of the plaintiff forced her resignation. In holding that intentional infliction of emotional distress occurred, even without proof of physical injury or touching, the court observed that "retaliatory behavior takes the case far beyond the ambit of insults and demeaning remarks."[43]

## Invasion of Privacy

The tort of *invasion of privacy* usually includes the element of publication; however, in sexual harassment cases, courts focus on intrusion and interference with the employee's right of privacy. For example, in one case a supervisor's conduct in making obscene phone calls to a plaintiff at her home and at work, as well as demeaning sexual comments about her, constituted an invasion of privacy. The court noted in that case that the type of invasion of privacy involved was "within the rubric of intrusion, a tort recognized in the District of Columbia." This tort does not include the publication of information; it focuses on interference with plaintiff's right to be left alone.[44]

## Wrongful Discharge

Plaintiffs also often include a common law claim for *wrongful discharge,* asserting that their discharge was in violation of a well-defined public policy inherent in antidiscrimination statutes and the state and federal Constitution. Generally, if an employee can establish that his or her termination was in retaliation for the exercise of a right recognized as public policy, the employer may be liable for compensatory and punitive damages. For example, if an employee can establish that he or she was terminated for pursuing a worker's compensation claim, a right established by state statute, the employer will be liable for wrongfully discharging the employee in violation of legislatively established public policy.

## CONCLUSION

In summary, failure to both know the law and appreciate and comply with the obligations imposed by laws can result in substantial liability for an employer. Consequently, it is imperative that management and supervisors be well trained in how to, first, avoid discriminatory practices and, second, effectively deal with employees who believe they have been discriminated against. Well-trained management and supervisory personnel are the keys to the successful operation of any business and to avoiding employment-related discrimination complaints.

## N O T E S

1. 42 U.S.C. Sec. 2000e et seq.
2. 42 U.S.C. Sec. 1981.
3. 42 U.S.C. Sec. 1983/1985.
4. 29 U.S.C. Sec. 225.
5. 29 U.S.C. Sec. 621 et seq.
6. 29 U.S.C. Sec. 701 et seq.
7. 42 U.S.C. 12-101 et seq.
8. Pub. L. 103-3.
9. See 42 U.S.C. 2000e(a) and 29 U.S.C. Sec. 23(d), respectively.
10. 411 U.S. 792 (1973).
11. See Texas Dept. of Community Affairs v. Burdine, 450 U.S. 248 (1981).
12. Meritor Savings Bank v. Vinson, 477 U.S. 57, 40 F.E.P. Cases 1822 (1986); Barnes v. Costle, 561 F.2d 983 (D.C. Cir. 1977); Tomkins v. Public Service Elec. & Gas Co., 568 F.2d 1044, 16 F.E.P. Cases 22 (3rd Cir. 1977); Garber v. Saxon Business Products, Inc., 552 F.2d 1032, 15 F.E.P. Cases 344 (4th Cir. 1977); Miller v. Bank of America, 600 F.2d 211, 20 F.E.P. Cases 462 (9th Cir. 1979); Henson v. City of Dundee, 682 F.2d 897, 29 F.E.P. Cases 787 (11th Cir. 1982); Simmons v. Lyons, 746 F.2d 265, 36 F.E.P. Cases 410 (5th Cir. 1984); Katz v. Dole, 709 F.2d 251, 31 F.E.P. Cases 1521 4th Cir. 1983); Rabidue v. Osceola Refining Co., 805 F.2d 611 (6th Cir. 1986) cert. denied 481 U.S. 1041.
13. 29 CFR §1604.11(a).
14. Meritor Savings Bank v. Vinson, 477 U.S. 57, 40 F.E.P. Cases 1822 (1986); Miller v. Bank of America, 600 F.2d 211, 20 F.E.P. Cases 462 (9th Cir. 1979); Barnes v. Costle, 561 F.2d 983 (D.C. Cir. 1977); Williams v. Civiletti, 487 F.Supp. 1387, 22 F.E.P. Cases 251 (D.D.C. 1980); Heelan v. Johns-Manville Corp., 451 F.Supp. 1382, 20 F.E.P. Cases 251 (D. Colo., 1978); Tomkins v. Public Service Elec. & Gas Co., 568 F.2d 1044, 16 F.E.P. Cases 22 (3rd Cir. 1977); Garber v. Saxon Business Products, Inc., 552 F.2d 1032, 15 F.E.P. Cases 344 (4th Cir. 1977); Ambrose v. U.S. Steel Corp., 39 F.E.P. Cases 35 (N.D.Cal. 1985); King v. Palmer, 778 F.2d 878, 39 F.E.P. Cases 877 (D.C. Cir. 1985); Christoforou v. Rider Truck Rental, 668 F.Supp. 294, 51 F.E.P. Cases 98 S.D.N.Y. 1987); Davis v. Utah Power & Light Co., 53 F.E.P. Cases 1332 (D. Utah 1990).
15. Meritor Savings Bank v. Vinson, 477 U.S. 57, 40 F.E.P. Cases 1155 (D.C. Cir 1981).
16. Harris v. Forklift Systems, Inc., 111 S.Ct. 367 (1993).
17. See, e.g., Bundy v. Jackson, 641 F.2d 934, 24 F.E.P. Cases 1155 (D.C. Cir. 1981).
18. Harris v. Forklift Systems, Inc., 114 C. Ct. 367 (1993).

19. Cline v. General Electric Credit Auto Lease, 748 F.Supp. 650, 54 F.E.P. Cases 419 (N.D. Ill. 1990); Ellison v. Brady, 924 F.2d 872, 54 F.E.P. Cases 1346 (9th Cir. 1991).
20. 29 C.F.R. §1604.11(b).
21. Huebschen v. Department of Health and Social Services, 547 F.Supp. 1168, 32 F.E.P. Cases 1521 (W.D. Wis. 1982), reversed and remanded for further proceedings, 716 F.2d 1167 (7th Cir. 1983).
22. See, e.g., Joyner v. AAA Cooper Transportation, 597 F.Supp. 537, 36 F.E.P. Cases 1644 (M.D. Ala. 1983). Title VII prohibitions of sexual harassment extend to homosexual as well as heterosexual conduct. Wright v. Methodist Youth Services, 511 F.Supp. 307, 25 F.E.P. Cases 563 (N.D. Ill. 1981), finding a cognizable claim under Title VII for an alleged termination of an employee who refused homosexual advances from his supervisor; Barlow v. Northwestern Memorial Hospital, 30 F.E.P. Cases 233 (D.C. Ill. 1980), holding that allegations by female employee that she was terminated for refusing to submit to her female supervisor's demands for sexual favors stated a cause of action under Title VII.
23. See, e.g., Carreno v. IBEW Local No. 226, 54 F.E.P. Cases 81 (D.Ka. 1990).
24. See, e.g., William v. Civiletti, 487 F.Supp. 1387 22 F.E.P. Cases 1311 (D.D.C. 1980).
25. 29 C.F.R. §1604.11(g). See also Toscona v. Nimmo, 570 F. Supp, 1197, 32 F.E.P. Cases 1401 (D. Del. 1983).
26. Tindall v. Housing Authority, 762 F. Supp. 259 55 F.E.P. Cases 22 (W.D. Ark. 1991).
27. Kouri v. Liberian Services, 55 F.E.P. Cases 124 (E.D. Vs. 1991).
28. Wensheimer v. Rockwell Intl. Corp., 54 F.E.P. Cases 828 (M.D.Fla. 1990).
29. 29 C.F.R. §1604.11(c).
30. Meritor Savings Bank v. Vinson, 477 U.S. 57, 40 F.E.P. Cases 1822 (1986); Henson v. City of Dundee, 682 F.2d 897, 29 F.E.P. Cases 787 (11th Cir. 1982); Horn v. Duke Homes of Windsor Mobile Homes, 755 F.2d 599 (7th Cir. 1985); Miller v. Bank of America, 600 F.2d 211, 20 F.E.P. Cases 462 (9th Cir. 1979); Barnes v. Costle, 561 F.2d 983 (D.C. Cir. 1977); Davis v. Utah Power & Light Co., 53 F.E.P. Case 1332 (D. Utah 1990).
31. Meritor Savings Bank v. Vinson, 477 U.S. 57, 40 F.E.P. Cases 1822 (1986).
32. Henson v. City of Dundee, 682 F.2d 897, 29 F.E.P. Cases 787 (11th Cir. 1982). See also Davis v. Western-Southern Life Ins. Co., 34 F.E.P. Cases 97 (N.D. Ohio 1984); Katz v. Dole, 709 F.2d 251, 31 F.E.P. Cases 1521 (4th Cir. 1983); Ferguson v. E.I. duPont de Nemours and Co., 560 F.Supp. 1172, 31 F.E.P. Cases 795 (D. Del. 1983); Coley v. Consolidated Rail Corp. 561 F.Supp. 645, 34 F.E.P. Cases 129 (D.C. Mich. 1982); Robson v. Eva's Super Market, 538 F.Supp. 857, 30 F.E.P. Cases 1212 (N.D. Ohio 1982); Henderson v. Pennwalt Corp., 704 P.2d 1256, 55 F.E.P. Cases 231 (Wash. App. 1985).
33. Jeppsen v. Wunnicke, 611 F.Supp. 78, 37 F.E.P. Cases 994 (D. Alaska 1985); Ambrose v. U.S. Steel Corp., 39 F.E.P. Cases 30 (N.D. Cal. 1985); Andresen v. McDonnell Douglas Corp., 55 F.E.P. Cases 525 (D. Utah 1991).
34. 29 C.F.R. §1604.11(d). See also Baker v. Weyerhaeuser Co., 903 F.2d 1342, 52 F.E.P. Cases 1872 (10th Cir. 1990) and Nash v. Electrospace, Inc., Case No. 93-1450 (5th Cir. December 17, 1993).
35. Guess v. Bethlehem Steel Corp., 913 F.2d 463, 53 F.E.P. Cases 1547 (7th Cir. 1990).
36. Bell v. St. Regis Paper Co., 425 F.Supp. 1126, 16 F.E.P. Cases 1429 (N.D. Ohio 1976).
37. Harris v. Forklift Systems, Inc., 114 S.Ct. 367 (1993).
38. 29 C.F.R. §1604.11(d)(e)(f).
39. Ellison v. Brady, 924 F.2d 872, 54 F.E.P. Cases 1346 (9th Cir. 1991).
40. Ferguson v. E.I. duPont Nemours and Co., 560 F.Supp.1172, 11 F.E.P. Cases 12 (D.C. Mich. 1982).
41. Barrett v. Omaha Nat'l Bank, 726 F.2d 424, 35 F.E.P. Cases 593 (8th Cir. 1984).
42. Crimm v. Missouri Pacific R. Co., 750 F.2d 703, 36 F.E.P. Cases 883 (8th Cir. 1984).
43. Shaffer v. National Can Corp., 565 F.Supp. 909, 34 F.E.P. Cases 172 (E.D.Pa. 1983).
44. Rogers v. Loews' L'Enfant Plaza Hotel, 526 F.Supp. 523, 29 F.E.P. Cases 828 (D.D.C. 1981).

# C H A P T E R 10

# Risk Management

Cathy K. Avdevich

**T**o understand the role of risk management in the health care delivery system, it is imperative to understand the terminology. *Risk management,* as defined by the Federation of American Hospitals Malpractice Subcommittee is the system for

> the identification, analysis and evaluation of risks and the selection of the most advantageous method for treating it. This is essentially synonymous to: Safety and Loss Prevention, Total Loss Control, Loss Control Management, etc. A risk management program should be a totally integrated program involving employee safety, patient safety, visitor safety, fire safety, security—in other words, a total-process safety program.[1]

This definition is as accurate in 1994 as when it was written in 1977. However, there are additional terms relevant to the management of risk and safety.

*Professional medical liability* is the risk management buzzword of the nineties, once known as medical negligence or malpractice. This new term more clearly defines the outcome of the risk event. Although the name for the event has not changed, negligence or malpractice is still the underlying risk issue. For example, when appropriate care is not given, medical negligence or malpractice may be the risk issue, but the responsible party or parties are liable for their conduct. The outcome of this example identifies the professional medical liability.

It is important for each facility to identify individuals who have the responsibility of reviewing actions that may pose a potential risk to that institution. Therefore, it is necessary to identify the purpose or goals for risk management and to identify by example how risks could occur.

## THE ROLE OF RISK MANAGEMENT

Risk management plays an important role in maintaining quality patient care while conserving the institution's financial resources. Elements that affect the risk management process include the incident, the loss potential, and the cost. An *incident* is any happening that is not consistent with the routine care of a particular patient. Every incident does not have the same outcome, but all incidents should be evaluated in terms of loss potential. Although not all incidents result in injury or damage, all incidents should be investigated.

*Loss potential* refers to any activity that costs the facility money or its good name (reputation). Cost to the facility could be related to additional charges for care of the patient which may be unrecoverable. For example, a patient comes into the department because of abdominal pain. While on the x-ray table, the patient's finger is cut or smashed by the bucky tray. In most cases, the facility has a policy and procedure to follow in the event of an injury to a patient. This policy may be interpreted by an employee to mean that the facility "takes care" of the patient any time the patient is injured in the facility. The injury requires a radiograph of the injured finger, sutures, bandages, medication to treat a possible infection, and the care of a physician and/or the emergency room. These charges may or may not be covered by the patient's insurance.

Due to the nature of the injury and because of comments made by the employee, the patient may feel that it is not his or his insurance company's responsibility to pay for this injury. Although the facility may be responsible for costs incurred for the immediate treatment, there is a potential long-term risk which may not be apparent on first glance.

What at first blush appears to be a small incident with relatively few costs has the potential to become a big problem. In addition to the facility being required to pay for initial treatment, the facility may be expected to take care of additional costs incurred. For example, the patient is unable to work until the stitches are removed; the patient is in advertising and has to give up being in a hand lotion commercial; a tendon is injured and reconstructive surgery is required; the surgery left a scar and a plastic surgeon must be consulted. Compensating a patient for such losses may be financially very costly, and failure to cooperate may lead to poor customer and community relations.

## Responsibility for Loss

It is every facility's responsibility to determine what, if anything, will be done for someone who is injured in the facility. The risk management department is responsible for establishing policies and procedures. After developing the procedures, all employees must be trained to follow appropriate actions for each particular type of incident. After this training, it is each employee's responsibility to know what should be said to the injured person regarding responsibility and liability.

## Developing Policies and Procedures

First, it is important to identify any situation that could pose a risk to the patient. Second, it is important to develop a method of practice to limit the potential risks to patients.

The role of risk management is to review all incidents that pose a risk to patients, visitors, employees, medical staff, volunteers, and students while at a facility. The overall responsibility for risk management usually rests with one to three staff members in larger facilities but may be part of one person's job responsibilities in an office or clinic.

Regardless of the size of the facility or the size of the risk management team, the most effective risk management system empowers all employees to function as risk managers. When all employees recognize the purpose of risk management principles and practice those principles, the number of potential risks to a facility may be reduced.

It is not enough to simply review occurrences that pose risks, a risk management system must also track these occurrences and look for trends. Once a trend is defined, a corrective action plan must be designed and implemented. Followup of the corrective action is essential. Evaluation of trends after the corrective action plan is implemented will either demonstrate the effectiveness of the plan or identify the need for modification and continued study.

## Investigation of Incidents

To understand the impact that incidents can have on liability for the facility, it is important to establish a method to investigate and evaluate the potential of each incident.

The investigation procedure for incidents may vary significantly based on the incident or even the facility's protocol, however, this phase is important and must be completed as systematically as possible. In most cases, the investigation begins at the department level. The manager or his or her designee reviews the incident report, talks with the staff involved, and makes notes as to what action, if any, needs to be taken. The manager then forwards the report to the risk manager for additional review. The risk manager reviews the report and determines if followup action is needed. Followup may include continuing the investigation, tracking the incident, or contacting other departments for additional information. In some cases, the risk manager will seek legal advice or advice from the insurance company.

One of the most important points of an investigation is the determination of whether the care rendered to the patient met the Standard of Care. Each separate incident may involve the review of the patient's chart, department records, and the employee's scope of practice. In addition, it must be determined whether the facility's policies and procedures were followed and that all of the necessary documentation is available. The review of policies and procedures may include both department-specific and facilitywide manuals. It should also be noted that, if it appears that the incident may go to litigation, all documents used in the investigation must be preserved. For example, if an incident occurred in 1993, the policies and procedures in effect on the date of the incident will be the documents requested for trial preparation.

The risk manager in larger facilities is usually responsible for reporting to the board of trustees, the administrative staff, and the safety committee. Obviously, this would be somewhat different in smaller facilities, clinics, or doctor's offices. In these settings, the office manager may be appointed to fulfill these duties. Regardless of the size of the facility, someone needs to be designated as the risk manager, and communication of activities needs to be reported to administration.

## Claims Prevention

Claims prevention and reducing the amount of claims against the facility are other important duties for the risk manager. Although it is the responsibility of the risk manager to identify risks that lead to potential claims, the task of claims reduction is also a component of the duties of the safety committee, the administration, and all facility staff.

Methods used to heighten staff awareness of safety policies and procedures are extremely effective in claim reduction. Two of the more common methods to increase awareness include additional education and stronger communication throughout the facility. The use of interdisciplinary committees or events may also increase the awareness of what happens in other departments.

In addition, adoption of the philosophy by all employees that it is easier to prevent incidents than to defend claims may also lead to claim reduction. Preventing incidents is a proactive response, whereas the tendency is to be reactive. The concept of being proactive rather than reactive is another challenge for the health care professional in the nineties.

## Communication

Most health care professionals rarely consider the types of risks that are inherent in each facility. One reason that may explain such lack of consideration is that health care professionals may not be aware of the outcome of incidents. For example, one might know that a patient fell in the department. The employee follows the procedure for reporting the incident and submits the report to the appropriate person. However, there may be no followup with or feedback to the person making the original report. If communication goes only in one direction, the originator may assume that there were no negative outcomes. This assumption may lead staff to believe that there are little or no risks in the department or facility. Be assured that every health care facility has a risk potential, and the risks are as many and as varied as there are people you work with every day. Each facility must have a mechanism for gathering data to determine what risks pose a liability to that facility.

## Risk Analysis

Risks can be divided into several categories, including risks to patients, to employees, to medical staff, and to others, including students, visitors, and volunteers. The following list may be used as a guide in determining which of these risks may be present and therefore may affect the facility's liability.

### Risks Related to Patients

Although more incidents take place in nursing departments, diagnostic imaging and radiation therapy departments have their fair share. One major issue to consider is that patients usually will not bring a lawsuit against an institution solely because of an injury. Patients often sue because they are angry at the caregivers and the way they were treated. Calling a person "honey" or "sweetie" may not be cause for a lawsuit, but if these terms anger the patient and the patient is subsequently injured, there is a greater likelihood that the patient's first response will be, "I'll sue."

Potential problem areas related to patients include the worst-case scenario of risk: death. While not a common occurrence, there have been incidents of death related to contrast media, equipment failure, and inappropriate use of drugs during a procedure. Spinal injuries resulting in paralysis can result from inappropriate manipulation of a patient with a spinal injury or from removal of a cervical collar without authorization.

Patient injury may occur when a patient falls due to slips on spilled liquid or trips over haphazardly placed equipment, electrical cords, and dropped items. Postural (orthostatic) hypotension has been associated with patient falls. Injuries to a patient may also occur during the course of a procedure. Bowel perforation may occur when barium enemas are not performed in the prescribed manner. Hips may be fractured when an unattended patient falls from a table or during transfer from chair or gurney to a table.

High-risk patients pose additional problems because age, level of understanding, level of consciousness, and medication complications may result in various types of injury, although falls are the most common cause of injury associated with these patients.

Failure to follow appropriate radiation protection measures, such as not providing shielding, failing to ascertain if there is a possibility of pregnancy, overexposing a patient because of examining the wrong patient, exposing the incorrect part of the body, or repeating films because of poor technique or positioning, are all situations that may result in injury to a patient and liability for the health care facility.

Breach of confidentiality injuries have occurred when an AIDS patient's medical information was discussed out of context or inappropriately or inadvertently offered to individuals not providing care to the patient. Other defamation of character claims have arisen when negative and untrue comments about a physician or coworker were spread throughout a facility.

## Risks to Employees

Although work-related injuries and illnesses make up a wide variety of potential risks to employees, as indicated in studies by OSHA, most injuries and illnesses to health care employees fall into relatively few categories. These risks are usually associated with employee failure to use proper techniques or protective devices and should be evaluated as such.

One method for gathering information on work-related employee injuries and illnesses would be to study the OSHA 200 Log. This is a report that must be posted at the work site annually during the month of February. The risk manager, employee health nurse, or human resources department are usually responsible for gathering data and maintaining the reports.

The following areas are most often associated with risk potential for employees: injury, including back injury; extremity injury, such as strains and sprains; needlesticks and sharps, with exposure to illnesses such as hepatitis and HIV; as well as multiple chemical sensitivities syndrome, more commonly known as darkroom disease.

Each facility must determine the appropriateness of the list and should add or change the categories as indicated by the occurrences reported.

## Medical Staff Risks and Issues

Medical staff are also at risk when involved in the delivery of health care services. In cases when the physician is not an employee of the facility, the risks may be attributed to activities on site and involvement in the overall process of patient care. The physician may be at risk from the actions of others and may be as susceptible to injury and illness as the employees. When the physician has an ownership interest in the facility, the risks may be multiplied, since the physician is the employer as well as the caregiver.

Medical staff issues are usually handled through a committee process or by a quality management department; however, the risk manager may serve as a liaison between the employees and medical staff through the incident reporting system. The following risk issues related to medical staff are based on professional publications from a variety of sources and should not be used as an absolute guide. Each facility should determine the appropriateness of the categories based on the activities and risks associated with the practice and the range of services offered.

The greatest physician risks are associated with incorrect diagnosis related to quality of radiographs, loss of radiographs, and failure to maintain original radiographs, and injuries from needlesticks and sharps and slips, trips, or falls.

## Risks to Others: Students, Visitors, and Volunteers

Risk to others is probably the most difficult area for risk managers to handle. Health care employees have been trained to care for patients and have been taught safety procedures for personal protection. The medical staff has a similar experience during educational preparation and through communication with the facility personnel. Students, visitors, and volunteers, however, usually have little or no training in policies and procedures required by the facility and often are under the impression that it is the facility's responsibility to care for them in the event of injury or illness. Actually, this perception may be further exacerbated by employees who also believe that these individuals have the same rights as patients and employees. It is up to the facility to review potential risks in this category and make employees aware of how these incidents should be handled.

The risks most commonly associated with students, visitors, and volunteers include injuries from slips, trips, or falls, and exposure to illness such as HIV and hepatitis.

## Equipment Risks and Issues

Risks and safety issues related to equipment are addressed by the Safe Medical Devices Act of 1990, which is covered in another chapter of this text. All health care employees should have a basic understanding of the components of this law. Equipment that malfunctions must be taken out of service immediately, and all packaging should be secured so that the investigating team has the information necessary to complete the investigation.

Although equipment malfunction may not be common, it does occur. User errors, on the other hand, while generally more common, may not always be reported, and therefore there may be no investigative procedures implemented and no corrective measures taken. It is important to understand that all employees must be comfortable and proficient with the equipment as well as the procedures that they perform.

## EMPLOYEE RESPONSIBILITY FOR RISK MANAGEMENT

While each facility needs an individual who has the authority and the responsibility to manage risk, it is essential that each employee also be involved in the process.

The employee's role in risk management is to follow department and facility policies and procedures, be aware of safety issues, and report hazardous conditions immediately. If an employee sees an accident, he or she should assess the situation, call for assistance, follow the policies and procedures of the facility, and always use common sense.

Until or unless an employee is involved in an investigation or legal action, potential risk may seem to be separate from his or her job duties. However, professional medical liability, loss prevention, and risk management must be a concern of all health care professionals.

## PUBLIC CONCERNS

Patient perceptions of radiation or health care in general are often related to what they read and what they hear. While it is important to remember that you can't believe everything you read, most people tend to believe the news, especially if the news is bad or if that person experienced something similar. Recent headlines have included stories on radiation experiments from the forties and fifties that are affecting the nineties and that the government knew about the tests. In the past, news headlines have covered reports of lawsuits and the settlements given for various incidents in the health care setting. All concerns that affect the public have an impact on the health care professional. Often, the patient questions the safety of the examination or the safety of radiation. These questions must be addressed with accurate and current information to reduce the patient's anxieties. To further illustrate the variety of news reported to the public, a brief list of headlines from one city's newspaper was gathered and is printed in the appendix.

## CONCLUSION

All health care facilities, regardless of size or structure, have inherent risks that can result in loss. Employee awareness and training as well as strong lines of communication are necessary to limit the potential for liability. Having a well-organized risk management program is the best method to control loss while providing for the safety and care of everyone in a health care facility.

## N O T E S

1. Federation of American Health Systems, *Risk Management Manual* (Little Rock, AR: Federation of American Hospitals, 1977).

## B I B L I O G R A P H Y

Harpster, Linda M., and Veach, Margaret S. *Risk Management Handbook for Health Care Facilities.* Chicago: American Hospital Publishing, 1990.
"Inadequate Fire Training Basis of $778,000 Lawsuit." *Biomedical Safety & Standards,* sample issue (Brea, CA: Quest Publishing Company, 1993).
Joint Commission on Accreditation of Healthcare Organizations. *Accreditation Manual for Hospitals.* Chicago: JCAHO, 1990–1993.
Kuntz, Larisa A. "Medical Negligence." *RT Image Radiographic Journal,* 6 January 1992.
McIntire, Suzanne. "Assault and Battery in Radiology." *RT 101. Wavelength* 4, no. 5 (February 1993).
Melbin, Jodi E. "Sedating the Pediatric Patient." *RT Image Radiographic Journal,* 19 October 1992.

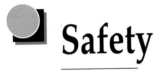

# Safety

Cathy K. Avdevich

**S**afety programs are an important component of all health care environments. While most hospital imaging department personnel are familiar with the safety policies and procedures of the facility, there are many technologists who work in other types of health care settings, which have few if any written safety procedures in place. Safety issues must be recognized in all health care settings, and safety programs should be developed regardless of the size or structure of the facility.

Developing an effective and efficient safety program requires the cooperation of the administration and the staff. Policies and procedures must be drafted in accordance with federal, state, and local regulations and analyzed in light of the specific needs of the facility.

## THE PROGRAM

An efficient safety program developed for the entire institution will generally include

1. Hazard identification and control
2. Written policies and procedures
3. Administrative/management support
4. Employee involvement
5. Employee training
6. Periodic inspections
7. Record keeping
8. A plan for enforcement of safety rules and regulations
9. When the facility has multiple departments, a safety committee

## Hazard Identification and Control

Safety begins with the recognition of all conditions that pose a risk in each facility. Hazard identification must be addressed as a systematic process. Development and use of a safety checklist is an effective method for identifying hazards. To create a checklist, at least two employees should complete a walkthrough of the department to observe working conditions and identify potential problems (see Appendix D–2).

In addition to the checklist, employee reports and suggestions may also identify actual and potential hazards. Review of equipment maintenance records may also be used to detect malfunctions and user errors that may have a direct impact on safety. Tracking incidents to determine trends related to safety is another mechanism used to identify hazards.

Once identified, hazards should be evaluated to determine how serious the problem may be. A corrective action plan should be developed and implemented, starting with the most potentially serious hazard and continuing until all issues are addressed. All occupations have some related hazards, and individual facilities will have a variety of potentially hazardous conditions. Federal guidelines concerning workplace safety, adopted and enforced by OSHA and other agencies, refer to potential hazards in diagnostic imaging and therapy departments (see Appendix D–3).

Two current hazards involving medical imaging departments center around the darkroom. First, the EPA has identified silver, found in used fixer, as a hazardous material with a federal limit for disposal of 5 ppm per liter. This means that the concentration of silver must be below five parts per million per liter in used fixer before being released into the waste stream. Some states, such as Kentucky,[1] accept the federal guidelines, while other states may be more strict. The second hazard also centers around chemicals found in the darkroom; however, this hazard deals with chemical sensitization to the processing chemicals, most often caused by poor ventilation. In 1992, articles in *RT Image*[2] labeled this sensitization "Darkroom disease." While the ventilation system in most larger facilities may reduce such incidents, staff at doctors' offices and clinics may be at greater risk. To best determine if there is a potential problem, the ventilation system should be checked, and the manufacturer of the chemicals should be consulted to advise on the appropriate number of air exchanges per hour based on room size.

The entire process of hazard identification and control related to chemicals should be governed by the facility's hazard communication policy. This policy is sometimes known as OSHA's right-to-know law.[3]

## Written Policies and Procedures

Written policies and procedures, supported by administration and management and followed by employees, will improve safety in a facility.

The safety of patients, employees, visitors, and property should be a major objective for all institutions.

Policies and procedures must be written to comply with all federal, state, and local laws for safety and health. A careful review of pertinent federal regulations will demonstrate the kinds of policies that must be followed by all facilities (see Appendix D–1). State and local laws should also be analyzed by each department or clinic when determining how to draft and implement safety policies and procedures.

While many state and local laws reflect the use of federal requirements, some state and local governments choose to have more stringent regulations. To be in compliance of the law, each facility must meet the most restrictive regulation.

Often hospitals are accredited by the Joint Commission on Accreditation of Healthcare Organizations (JCAHO), but not all medical imaging facilities seek this approval. Whether a facility chooses to meet these standards or not, the intent of DR.2.2.3, DR.2.2.6 of the accreditation guidelines could be used to establish a list of policies and procedures related to safety.[4]

## Policy and Procedure Recommendations

Regardless of the size or nature of the facility, every provider of health care services should develop a series of policies and procedures which address questions of safety that may arise in the particular setting. Suggested topics for general safety-related policies and procedures include but are not limited to the following:

1. Fire safety
2. Electrical safety
3. Hazardous materials and waste management, to include
   a. The hazard communication standard
   b. Generating/disposing hazardous materials
4. Occurrence reporting and loss prevention due to injury
5. Emergency codes, to include
   a. External disasters
   b. Internal disasters
   c. Evacuation procedures
   d. Cardiopulmonary arrest
6. Back safety
7. Infection control
8. Patient transport and lifting techniques

Specific departmental concerns should also be addressed by policy and procedures. Diagnostic imaging and radiation oncology departments contain equipment and materials that are very hazardous and must be maintained in a controlled environment. Therefore, it is imperative that policies and procedures to address these issues be drafted by the department management in conjunction with department personnel and the facility's risk manager or safety officer.

Issues affecting departmental safety include but are not limited to

1. Equipment management, to include
   a. Equipment use
   b. Equipment safety
   c. Safe Medical Devices Act (SMDA)
2. Radiation safety, to include
   a. Patient protection
   b. Personnel protection
   c. Protection of others
   d. Quality control procedures (Quality control procedures include all aspects of image production that reduce the dose of radiation to patients, personnel, and others.)
3. Safe practice for use of radiopharmaceuticals
4. Safe practice for use of a radiation source (therapy)
5. Immobilization techniques

## Administrative/Management Support

Inherent in the philosophy of most health care facilities is provision of a safe environment for patients, employees, and others. Those facilities under the review process by the JCAHO are required to meet the standards for Plant, Technology, and Safety Management (PTSM). The JCAHO-related standards require that the governing body of the facility support the establishment and maintenance of an effective safety program. Whether the facility accepts the guidelines published in the JCAHO Accreditation Manuals for Hospitals or not, the standards are an excellent guide for the establishment of a safety program. When the governing body, administration, and management of a facility accept responsibility for safety, the support for safety education programs for employees will be more readily available.

## Employee Involvement

Employee safety involvement becomes more apparent as the level of awareness and education increases. When employees picture themselves as part of the process, safety procedures are more likely to be practiced. One method for improving involvement is to provide safety information in each departmental meeting. Having at least one person from the department serving on the facility's multidisciplinary safety committee and bringing information back to department personnel is another way to increase safety awareness. Mandating annual safety education programs would be another method for increasing awareness and safety practices in the department. Examples of mandated programs include fire safety, infection control, and back safety. Managers should also evaluate all incidents that involve safety issues and discuss in department meetings ways to reduce repeat incidents. Group discussion of potential and actual safety incidents is an effective way to identify and avoid risks in the facility (see Figure 11–1).

## Employee Training

Safety training is an integral part of employee education and training. The education may take place as a facilitywide training program or may be department specific. Based on the facility's policies and procedures, safety training should be based on competencies and written objectives which provide the learner with a list of expectations. The type of safety programs that should be offered will vary from facility to facility, but programs that are important in any health care environment are facility-wide safety issues, such as fire safety or infection control, as well as department-specific issues like electrical safety for imaging equipment. The following sample in-service programs are intended to be used as a guide to assist facilities in developing their own safety programs.

### Fire Safety Procedures

*Purpose:* Fire in any environment may result in loss of life. In a health care setting, the employee must consider how to act or react in all situations. To be prepared in the event of fire or smoke, the employee must be familiar with the procedures to follow to either fight a small fire or evacuate the facility.

To be appropriately trained, the employee must be able to meet the following objectives.

*Objectives:*

Upon completion of this program, the employee will:

1. State the acronym used when a fire occurs and describe the action needed for each letter of the word.
2. State the acronym used when a fire extinguisher is to be used and describe the action needed for each letter of the word.
3. Given a list of do's and don't's, determine what action would be appropriate for fire safety.
4. Discuss the need for evacuation of patients, staff, and others in the event of a fire.

The following sample outline may serve as a guide to establish a presentation on fire safety. In larger facilities, the safety officer often presents this material. However, this sample could be used by a member of a local fire department to train employees at a smaller facility.

## Educational Presentation Outline

1. Fire Safety
   a. RACE

   R — RESCUE persons from the area of the fire
   Feel doors for heat
   Know exit locations and fire compartments
   A — ACTIVATE alarm
   Call hospital operator/911/fire station
   C — CONTAIN/CONTROL the fire
   Close all doors and windows (It is important that doorstops, or wedges, not be used.)
   E — EXTINGUISH/EVACUATE
   1) Use a portable fire extinguisher (PASS)

   P — Pull the pin
   A — Aim at base of fire
   S — Squeeze the trigger
   S — Sweeping motion for the spray
   2) Evacuate the room, compartment, floor (horizontally, then vertically). Do *not* use the elevator

   b. Fire Safety Do's and Don't's
   DO:

   — Follow smoking regulations.
   — Store oxygen cylinders in designated storage areas.
   — Transport oxygen cylinders in the stand; do *not* carry by grasping the neck or valve of the cylinder or transport by laying cylinder on the stretcher or bed.
   — Store flammables in approved safety containers.
   — Ground equipment properly.
   — Check wires for frayed insulation and other defects.
   — Safety check or have safety checks done on all personal appliances (hairdryer, toaster).
   — Keep heat away from combustible materials.
   — Keep passageways free from obstruction and have them well marked.
   — Check fire doors to see that they open easily and close tightly.
   — Dispose of waste safely in approved, fire-resistant containers.

DON'T:

— Overload circuits.
— Run cords under rugs (avoid the use of extension cords when possible).

2. Fire Extinguishers

If the fire is extensive or threatening, evacuate the area.

If the fire is small and confined to a small area and you are trained in the use of a fire extinguisher, you may choose to fight the fire.

Be certain you have the appropriate extinguisher for the type of fire:

TYPE A — Use on wood, cloth, paper, or rubbish
TYPE B — Use on oil, paint, grease, or flammable liquids
TYPE C — Use on electrical equipment fires

A multipurpose fire extinguisher (ABC) can be used on all three types of fire.

Fire extinguishers require proper maintenance, and records should be maintained on each extinguisher which document the dates of inspection, recharge, and repair.

3. Fire Evacuation

It is important to evacuate the area of a fire to a safe place. This may mean to evacuate a room, a wing, a floor, or the entire facility. It is essential to have a well thought-out plan for evacuation. Fire barriers and smoke compartments should be identified, and exit signs must be posted. Large facilities probably have these safety standards in place, but all facilities need to be in compliance with fire safety rules and regulations. Most community fire departments will assist in the development of fire policies and procedures and will often assist with staff training in fire safety.

### Employee Injury Prevention

*Purpose:* A major goal of any facility is to provide quality care in the safest way possible. This includes safety not only for the patient but for the employee as well. To reduce the risk of injury, employees must recognize the potential for risk and the appropriate procedures to follow for each type of risk. To meet this goal, each employee must meet the following objectives.

*Objectives:*

Upon completion of this program, the employee will:

1. Identify two potential causes of employee injury.
2. Discuss rules for safe practice when using needles or sharps.

3. Discuss the appropriate sections in the facility's exposure control plan which addresses the rules for handling needles and sharps.
4. Discuss rules for safe practice when using chemicals.

To meet the objectives for employee injury prevention training, the following outline may be used. However, this sample is intended as a guide, and additional topics should be addressed as needed based on the injuries specific to the discipline and the facility.

### Educational Presentation Outline

1. Physical Injuries to Employees
   a. Needlestick/sharps injuries rules for safe practice include
      — Let falling objects fall. Do *not* grab for falling instruments or glassware.
      — Use safe handling techniques for uncapping needles. A slow, steady, two-hand technique allows for greater control. Watch the tip at all times. Do *not* bend, break, or recap* used needles.
      — Dispose of sharps immediately after use in specially designed and labeled containers. Do *not* overfill any container.
      — Do *not* reach into any container.
      — If a needlestick/sharp incident occurs, report the injury immediately and refer to the appropriate infection control policy and procedures.
   b. Chemical hazards involve a wide variety of risks. Know what chemical you are using by using the following guidelines:
      — Read the container label carefully. Do *not* use anything from an unmarked container. If the label is torn or illegible, replace it immediately.
      — Review the material safety data sheets (MSDS) for detailed information on the safety hazards and specific precautions for the safe use of the product.
      — Use proper handling techniques:
        (1) Follow only the approved method for mixing chemicals.
        (2) Ventilate the work area as recommended.
        (3) Always wear proper personal protective equipment.

---

*Recapping needles in special circumstances may be allowed, but a policy and procedure with all special circumstances must be in place in the exposure control plan described in the bloodborne pathogen standard. A description of special equipment or method must be included in the documentation.

---

1. It is your responsibility to alert others to danger.
2. No matter how long you have been on the job, it is your responsibility to ask questions whenever you have doubts.
3. If you cannot remove or repair a hazard yourself, report it to your supervisor immediately.
4. Prevention is the best cure for dermatitis. If you get chemicals on your hands, wash them immediately.
5. Find out who to contact if your equipment needs to be serviced. Do *not* make repairs yourself unless you are trained to do so.
6. Tripping hazards are common. Keep extension cords, phone lines, and other obstacles out of aisles and passageways.
7. Never handle electrical equipment if your skin or clothes are wet or damp.
8. Use caution whenever removing objects from high shelves or cabinets.
9. Clean up broken glass with a broom and dustpan, *not* your hands. Place broken glass in a puncture-proof container, and label the container so that others will not get cut.
10. Always wear the required personal protective equipment, even if the job will "only take a minute."
11. Safety is a full-time job. Pay attention to your surroundings and to what you are doing at all times. Don't take shortcuts.
12. Inspect equipment regularly. Equipment that needs service or repair must be tagged and removed from the area.
13. *Never* lift anything too heavy. Get help.
14. Obey all warning signs; they are there for your protection.

---

■ FIGURE 11–1   **SAMPLE SAFETY RULES AND REMINDERS**

— Use appropriate methods to dispose of chemicals:
  (1) Use and store chemicals in approved containers that are properly labeled.
  (2) Dispose of chemicals according to the guidelines for each chemical. Many chemicals cannot be poured into drains or sewers.

Safety training can also be accomplished by having written materials available for use in department meetings or as handouts that can be placed on department bulletin boards. A list of safety rules and reminders may serve as a training method using written materials. The list could be distributed in a meeting, and each employee could discuss what rule may need more explanation (Figure 11–1).

Training during a meeting should be well documented in the minutes for the meeting; it is also desirable for all employees to sign a form showing attendance.

## Periodic Inspections

All patient care areas in a facility should have a formal in-house safety inspection at least twice a year. When the facility is large enough to have a multidisciplinary safety committee, it is usually the committee's responsibility to complete these safety inspections. However, to increase awareness of safety needs in a department, it may be appropriate to appoint a group from the department to tour the area and make suggestions on a more frequent basis. Records of the inspection results should be maintained.

## Record Keeping

There are a number of documents that need to be maintained for departments of diagnostic imaging and therapeutic radiology. Depending on the nature of the documents and the agencies that may require documentation, a system needs to be implemented to ensure that appropriate records are maintained.

These records may include the dosimetry reports for all employees, the manifest for disposal of used fixer, or, as previously mentioned, the safety inspections for the department.

Since many records must be maintained for extended periods, storage of the materials may present a problem to an imaging or therapy department. Therefore, the facility should develop a system for preserving records. When inspections, such as safety surveys, are made, the department may be required to correct deficiencies. If corrective action is required, records of those activities should also be maintained.

## Enforcement of Rules and Regulations

Rules and regulations come from a variety of sources and should be adhered to as written. One method for determining compliance with the rules or regulations is to establish policies and procedures that address each issue. It is not enough, however, to have the appropriate policies and procedures unless the staff follows them. Therefore, regular in-service or department meetings should be held to update the staff on policy changes and implementation. At a minimum, an annual review of the policies and procedures is needed to determine compliance. Corrective action for all problems or issues must be both consistent and timely to be effective.

## Safety Committee

As mentioned in other sections of this chapter, a safety committee should be formed to establish, maintain, and evaluate the effectiveness of the safety program in each facility. The committee's structure will depend on the size and services offered in each facility. Whenever possible, the committee should have representatives from each discipline, as well as administrative representation. The safety committee should meet frequently and should communicate the activities that are being addressed. The effectiveness of the safety program and the safety committee's actions should be evaluated at least annually. The more effective the actions of the safety program, the more effective the risk prevention process will be.

## CONCLUSION

Safety is important for all health care providers. Having an effective safety program will reduce the risk of injury to patients, employees, and others. Employee involvement will strengthen the process. To ensure employee involvement, effective training programs and quality procedures for practice are essential. The goal must be to make safety a top priority for each facility. As safety increases, risk and liability decrease. Accepting this concept is one way to meet the requirements of continuous quality improvement.

## NOTES

1. OSHA Guidelines, 401 KAR 31:010, Title 401, ch. 31, 32.
2. Larisa A. Kuntz, "Help for Darkroom Disease," *RT Image,* 28 September 1992, 11, 22. See also related article, 31 August 1992.
3. Federal "Hazard Communication Standard," as administered by the U.S. Department of Labor, Occupational Safety and Health Administration (OSHA).
4. Joint Commission on the Accreditation of Healthcare Organizations, *Accreditation Manual,* 1994.

## REFERENCES

Bureau of National Affairs. *BNA's Health Care Facilities Guide.* Washington, D.C.: U.S. Government Printing Office, 1994.

*Coastal Healthcare. Medical Waste Handling.* Virginia Beach, Va.: Coastal Video Communications Corp., 1993

"Draft Guidelines for Preventing the Transmission of Tuberculosis in Health-Care Facilities." 2nd ed. Notice of Comment Period. Centers for Disease Control and Prevention, Department of Health and Human Services. Federal Register, 12 October 1993.

"Enforcement Policy and Procedures for Occupational Exposure to Tuberculosis." Memorandum for Regional Administrators. OSHA. 8 October 1993.

*Guideline for Handwashing and Hospital Environmental Control.* Atlanta: Centers for Disease Control, 1985 (NTIS no. PB85-923404/LL).

*Guideline for Infection Control in Hospital Personnel.* Atlanta: Centers for Disease Control, 1988 (NTIS no. PB85-923402/LL).

*Guideline for Isolation Precautions in Hospitals.* Atlanta: Centers for Disease Control, 1983 (NTIS no. PB85-923401).

Hodges, James. *Handling Hazardous Waste Materials.* Louisville, Ky.: Raynostix Corp., 1990.

Kelly, Jack. "AIDS Questions About Care?" *RT Image.* 29 November 1993.

Kuntz, Larisa A. "Darkroom Disease." *RT Image,* 31 August 1992.

Kuntz, Larisa A. "Health-Care Workers and HIV—Are CDC's New Guidelines Effective?" *RT Image,* 5 August 1991.

Kuntz, Larisa A. "HELP for Darkroom Disease." *RT Image,* 28 September 1992.

Loudin, Amanda. "Radiology's Part in Protecting Mother Earth." *RT Image,* 23 September 1991.

Lynch, Patricia, et al. "Implementing and Evaluating a System of Generic Infection Precautions: Body Substance Isolation." *American Journal of Infection Control* 18, no. 1 (February 1990).

Mehne, Carol. "CAUSE FOR CAUTION! Infectious-Disease Risk in the Workplace." *RT Image,* 29 November 1993.

Mehne, Carol. "AIDS, The Prevention Promise." *RT Image,* 29 November 1993.

Melbin, Jodi E. "What Price Environment?????" *RT Image,* 26 October 1992.

*Most Frequently Asked Questions Concerning the Bloodborne Pathogens.* OSHA. November 1992.

Occupational Safety and Health Administration. *Preamble to Bloodborne Pathogens Standard.* 56 Federal Register 64004.

Parkin, William P. *The Complete Guide to Environmental Law.* North Vancouver, Canada: STP Specialty Technical Publishers, 1993.

Piotti, Debora S. "The Three Rs of the EPA." *RT Image,* 12 July 1993.

"Recommendations for Preventing Transmission of Human Immunodeficiency Virus and Hepatitis B Virus to Patients During Exposure-Prone Invasive Procedures." *MMWR* 40, no. RR-8 (July 1991).

"Recommendations for Prevention of HIV Transmission in Health-Care Settings." *MMWR* 36, no. 2S (August 1987).

Stecher, Anna. "HIV in Nuclear Medicine; Questions Raised About Infection Control Policy." *RS Wavelength* 4, no. 9 (June 1993).

*Supervisor's Safety Meeting Handbook.* Madison, Conn.: Business & Legal Reports, Inc., 1993.

"Update: Universal Precautions for Prevention of Transmission of Human Immunodeficiency Virus, Hepatitis B Virus, and Other Bloodborne Pathogens in Health-Care Settings." *MMWR* 37, no. 24 (June 1988).

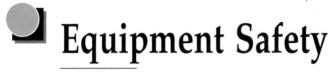

# Equipment Safety

Cathy K. Avdevich


**P**atient and personnel safety can hinge on the condition of the equipment used in the health care setting. The Safe Medical Devices Act of 1990 was implemented to protect individuals from faulty medical devices. Diagnostic imaging and therapeutic radiology personnel must understand both the global application of this act as well as the specifics affecting departments and clinics. Along with equipment failure and malfunction, products may be recalled when it has been determined that the equipment may harm the operator or the consumer.

## SAFE MEDICAL DEVICES ACT OF 1990 (SMDA)[1]

The Safe Medical Devices Act of 1990 (SMDA) requires that manufacturers and user facilities report to the Food and Drug Administration (FDA) deaths, serious injury, and serious illness attributed to medical devices. User facilities are defined as hospitals, nursing homes, outpatient treatment centers, and ambulatory surgical facilities. Physicians' offices and group practices that implant or distribute tracked devices are also regulated under the tracking rule. According to an *ECRI Advisory* publication, the "FDA has the authority under SMDA to conduct audits of medical device manufacturers regulated by the tracking rule."[2] The manufacturers are required to develop a method of tracking. "Because hospitals and other health care providers are a principal source of device tracking information, they naturally will be affected by the manufacturer's obligation to ensure the accuracy of their method."[3]

The SMDA is comprised of two major components: (1) adverse event reporting and (2) medical device tracking. Both aspects of the law must be understood and followed by user facilities.

## Adverse Event Reporting

The adverse event reporting portion of the law became effective November 28, 1991. However, upon implementation there was a great deal of confusion over which events to report and how they should be reported. To alleviate any confusion, in June 1993, the FDA announced the new Medical Products Reporting Program, "MedWatch."[4]

MedWatch was developed and implemented to simplify the process of reporting adverse events and product problems. The MedWatch reporting form is available in two versions: one for voluntary (Form 3500) and one for mandatory (Form 3500A) reporting (see Appendix E).

Form 3500 is to be used by health professionals for voluntary reporting of adverse events or product problems to manufacturers or to the FDA and will receive limited discussion in this text.

Form 3500A, the mandatory reporting version, must be used by user facilities, distributors, and manufacturers for all adverse events that are considered serious. The reportable events include the patient outcome involving death, a life-threatening condition, initial or prolonged hospitalization, disability, congenital anomaly, or required surgical or medical intervention to prevent permanent impairment or damage.[5]

## Medical Device Tracking

Medical device tracking went into effect on August 29, 1993. The purpose of this component is to ensure that manufacturers of tracked devices can locate and recall defective or dangerous devices and notify patients using them. The current list of devices to be tracked is subject to change as needed, and it is up to the facility to maintain an up-to-date list of the requirements of this law (see Appendix E). While it is important for the medical imaging professional to understand the content of a law, it is especially important to recognize that a tracking system must be put into effect, and the medical imaging professional must understand his or her responsibility for tracking to achieve compliance.

---

## IMPLEMENTING A SAFE MEDICAL DEVICES ACT COMPLIANCE PROGRAM

As with any system, it is important to assign responsibility for development, implementation, and evaluation of the process. The overall responsibility for SMDA is usually given to the facility's safety committee. The safety committee will then assign or appoint an individual or a small group to study the requirements and develop the process. The appointed individual or group will determine who will assume overall responsibility for managing the program. Together, these individuals will review current practices, as well as develop and implement policies and procedures. The procedure should include who reports to the manufacturer and who maintains the up-to-date list of trackable devices.

As a brief overview, the following program outline may be used as a checklist for setting up a compliance program for device tracking. However, each facility must take responsibility for complying with the intent of the law.

1. Assign overall responsibility.
2. Review current practices and identify changes or modifications needed to meet the requirements.
3. Develop policies and procedures.
4. Determine who reports to the manufacturer.
5. Determine who will maintain an up-to-date list of trackable devices.
6. Develop and implement appropriate staff training.
7. Evaluate the effectiveness of the program and make changes as needed.
8. Communicate activities to the appropriate administrative bodies.

As the system is developed and implemented, staff must become aware of the role they play in facility compliance with the Safe Medical Devices Act.

## EMPLOYEE AWARENESS

As demonstrated in the overview, different levels of awareness are necessary for facility staff. As a general guideline, training can be addressed at four levels: (1) general staff, (2) device operators, (3) the incident investigating team, and (4) user facility managers.[6]

General staff usually comprise the majority of staff and often need training only in the area of awareness of the law and the penalties for noncompliance. The second level, device operators, must, along with having an overall awareness of the law, take responsibility for reporting the occurrence, removing the device from use, and maintaining the security of the device and package for use in the investigation. The investigating team needs to have a complete understanding of the law and of the policies and procedures governing the investigative process. The team must know how to maintain materials and convey the outcome of the investigation to the managerial staff. Overall responsibility for facility compliance rests with the fourth group, the user facility managers. This group must meet the deadline for reporting as required in the regulation. Ultimately, the facility must determine which personnel belong in each category and what each group should be taught. The diversity of personnel in diagnostic and therapeutic medical imaging departments will determine which levels of education and responsibility will be necessary for the facility.

After implementation of the compliance program, an evaluation must be undertaken to determine the program's effectiveness. The evaluation results should be conveyed to the administrative staff.

Overall, each staff member should have at least a working knowledge of how this law affects health care. In addition to knowledge of the SMDA, staff should also be aware that the facility's management is involved in an equally important process related to products and devices: product recalls.

## PRODUCT RECALLS

Many Americans have been exposed to recall notices for automobiles, toys, or drug products. However, a large number of health care workers are not aware that their facility may be receiving notice of product recalls on a daily or at least monthly basis. As with many other activities in a facility, only a select few personnel are aware of the significance of this subject. Manufacturers notify facilities of problems with products so that each facility can take definitive action to reduce the risk of liability. It is imperative that the facility have an appropriate process to handle all recall notices. The most difficult aspect of the product recall process is determining who has received the recall notices. Once this dilemma has been solved, the facility must develop a system of communication between the individual who receives notice and the person or persons responsible for taking action. The most effective way of handling this problem is to assign responsibility to an individual or group, develop appropriate policies and procedures, educate the staff, and evaluate the process. The key to an effective system is education and communication. Each and every staff member should understand the process and the method for communicating necessary information to the appropriate person or group.

Both SMDA and product recall processes affect professionals in diagnostic and therapeutic medical imaging. The degree of impact depends on the role and responsibility of each professional. It is up to the professional and the department's management to determine what each staff member should know, while recognizing that all personnel need at least a working knowledge of what is required in the facility.

## Impact of SMDA and Product Recall on Medical Imaging

Depending on the length of time in the profession, many radiographers have little, if any, historical knowledge of problems related to injuries from medical equipment or products. There have, however, been many such occurrences.

As early as 1987, newspapers and magazines around the country reported adverse events related to devices and products. An example of one such report involved a cancer patient who was crushed by a cobalt machine. In an update report on this incident (15 October 1988), the hospital reported that the 3,400-pound arm of the machine "suddenly abruptly gave way as it was being lowered by the radiology technician using a hand-held control device."[7]

The injury from the faulty cobalt equipment was not an isolated event related to product and equipment incidents. The professional publication *RS Wavelength*[8] reported allergic reactions to latex and the need to develop new products to lessen the chance of adverse reactions.

In 1986, *People* magazine reported that a computer glitch caused severe injury and death to three cancer patients.[9] To compound the problem of the device malfunction in each of these cases, all three patients immediately complained of intense heat coming from the units. It appeared that no health care professional responded to the incident as an actual malfunction at the time of the patient complaint. Had a mechanism been in place, one or two of these injuries may have been avoided. The first incident occurred on June 4, 1985; the second occurred on March 21, 1986; and the third occurred 22 days later.

Another example of a documented event was reported in *RS Wavelength* in June 1993: "MRI Death Leads to Caution. . . ." The FDA issued a caution for ordering or performing MR scans on patients with an intracranial aneurysm clip.[10] At the time of this report, there was no way to determine which clips could be safely scanned.

These are just a few of the many reports from sources related to the discipline. There have likewise been many reports and product recalls concerning various types of contrast materials, other drugs used in examinations, products, and equipment used in the discipline.

## Field Corrections of Recalls

As reported in *Radiology & Imaging Letter,* one manufacturer is providing precautionary instructions for a linear accelerator that could cause a therapy overdose.[11] As noted in the recall, if not corrected, there is a potential for patients to receive ten times the dose required. In this same report, a drug company recalled certain kits for the preparation of a radiopharmaceutical because the reconstituted vial's physical appearance may not meet the description in the package insert.[12] In this same issue, other products were cited for a variety of reasons. The following examples are included to demonstrate the types and variety of products reported in just one publication. The first example identifies that the FDA has concluded that a breast transilluminator is not clinically effective for the diagnosis or detection of breast cancer or other breast abnormalities. In addition, one model was recalled because "the product labeling fails to bear adequate directions for use."[13] Two other examples identified the need for recalls or field corrections for both nuclear imaging systems and ultrasound systems software.[14] The final example identified a recall for mammography film due to possible artifacts that may be potentially misinterpreted by radiologists.[15]

A review of previous issues of *Radiology & Imaging Letter* revealed additional significant warnings. For example, in the May 1994 issue, three models of videobronchoscopes were recalled because static electricity discharge could cause a CCD chip failure.[16] This failure could lead not only to loss of the image, but could cause heating at the distal end. At the time of this report, however, no adverse incidents had occurred.

A second item in this edition reported that a company was conducting a field correction on an MRI phantom. According to this report, "the anatomical phantom used by technicians during quality assurance evaluation will malfunction with respect to evaluating left-right image reversal."[17]

While most reports listed in this publication appear to focus on radiation therapy, nuclear medicine, ultrasound, and mammography equipment, routine radiographic equipment is not exempt from recall. In the June 15, 1994, report, an image intensifier system positioning arm was recalled because of "an improper weldment on the arm structure for the image intensifier may crack and fall."[18] As indicated in this report, a company spokesperson told the newsletter staff that "the company issued a safety notice on the potential weld problem in February 1994" and stated, "We moved quickly to implement corrective action by sending out service engineers to inspect the small number of units involved for a problem weld on the support piece. If the weld was improper, that part of the system was replaced."[19] This account is an excellent example of the need for the manufacturer to respond to potential risks by instituting a corrective action plan. However, it should also serve as a model for health care facilities to have a system in place to respond to product recalls or potential risk situations in a timely manner.

Examples of product recalls, field corrections, and safety hazards identified in the previous section come from a limited source and within a limited time frame: one professional publication over a one-year period. This is a strong indication that there are many other potential problems that exist in the working environment.

One question that might be asked at this point is "How does each facility identify potential problems?" The best answer to this question is to begin to research the subject by gathering as much data as possible on what type of recalls the facility has received within the last three to five years. Following this department-specific research, identify any government departments (both federal and state) that have responsibility for product safety related to medical equipment and products. Additional sources may also include professional journals and publications as well as local newspapers and magazines.

## Warnings

In addition to SMDA and product recalls, other information related to devices or products may serve as a warning to the medical community. In May 1994, the FDA asked "manufacturers of contrast agents to place a boxed warning on the carton, vial, and package insert labeling for each iodinated contrast product (or concentration) that is not intended for intrathecal use."[20] This request from the FDA was initiated because of reports of misadministration that resulted in serious adverse events, such as convulsions, coma, and death. Included with this warning is the statement directed to the health care professional to "thoroughly familiarize themselves" with the package insert and the appropriate drug for the route of administration used. The health care professional is also encouraged by the FDA to report adverse events through the MedWatch program.

Another report in this bulletin made reference to the investigation of the safety of tattoos in the performance of MRI procedures. While the most common problem with tattoos is related to the exposure to blood-borne pathogens and sensitivity to the pigments used, there is now an additional risk. It appears that some of the pigments used in tattooing are made of metallic salts, such as iron oxide. This pigment may pose a risk to the patient having an MRI.[21] At present, this is still being investigated by the FDA. However, the agency is asking clinicians to report problems related to tattoos and MRI through the MedWatch program. In an article published in June 1993, a case study on a 26-year-old male having an MRI scan of his cervical spine reported a tattoo reaction to the effects of MRI.[22] None of the reactions listed in the study resulted in long-term effects, nor were they considered to be serious, but lack of reporting this event may have led to delay in a study by the FDA.

While not applicable under a discussion of either SMDA or product recalls, there is another category that must be addressed related to both equipment and products: user errors.

## USER ERRORS

Using equipment and products incorrectly or inappropriately is classified as *user error*. While SMDA and product recall focus on the manufacturer, user error is directly focused on the health professional. Historically, medical imaging professionals have laughingly told the patient that the processor "ate" the film or that the "patient must have moved" as a cover for a technical error. However, the technical error was often a result of user error. User errors may be the result of a variety of causes, such as inattention to details or rushing to finish the procedure. A more common type of user error, which most imaging professionals have yet to address, is the utilization of equipment or products without the education or experience needed for safe operation. For example, a new piece of equipment is brought to the department and the salesperson conducts in-service training to demonstrate how the equipment is to be used. The in-service may fail to include all personnel who may be responsible for using the equipment. To try to meet the needs of the personnel, one staff member may be selected to "show" how the equipment operates to the staff that were unable to attend the original in-service. While in the minds of management this may seem to be an appropriate method of training, it lacks an extremely important element. The missing element in this scenario is that the original staff member was shown how the equipment worked, but there was no mechanism to evaluate the competency of that individual prior to being asked to "train others." It must be management's responsibility to review how new equipment is introduced into a department, and it must be the responsibility of both management and each individual staff member to ascertain the competence level necessary for using all equipment and products and for performing all procedures in the facility.

User errors may result in a wide variety of injuries to both the patient and the worker. For example, as a result of increased back injuries from lifting, many facilities have adopted the use of back belts. Generally, the belts are passed out in a meeting, where everyone is told the same basic information about how the belt is to be used. What is often overlooked in this process is the fact that the belts need to be properly fitted and that the employee should be evaluated on the actual use of lifting techniques while wearing the back belt. A more common problem with the scenario is that the in-service is held once for everyone, but new employees, hired after the date of the in-service, may not be given the necessary instruction. Compounding the issue of back belt utilization to reduce injuries in the workplace, the National Institute for Occupational Safety and Health (NIOSH)[23] has issued a warning that in summary states that back belts may not help and may even do harm.

There are many other examples of potential problems related to user errors. Venipuncture is a current professional controversy, even though many technologists have been injecting contrast media for years. When injury occurs following an injection, the contrast media reaction is usually the focus of concern. While contrast media reaction may be the cause of some problems related to venipuncture, the actual technique used to place the needle may cause problems such as phlebitis in patients. Not all cases of phlebitis are caused by inappropriate venipuncture technique but some cases are directly related to poor technique, which is classified as a form of user error. According to a report in *Biomedical Safety & Standards*,[24] "Human Errors Key to Infusion-Related Lawsuits," "human error is often cited as the cause" for problems and lawsuits.

Additional examples of potential user error include

1. Overinflation of foley catheters and barium enema tip balloons.
2. Excessive force while inserting an enema tip.
3. Overdosage of medications and / or radiopharmaceuticals.
4. Filling syringes with two different types of drugs, such as alcohol in one syringe and contrast media in the other, and injecting the incorrect drug into the IV.
5. During surgery, a patient's leg comes in contact with the collimator, the leg is draped, and following surgery the collimator light is found to be on, resulting in second- and third-degree burns to the patient.
6. A foot rest, detached during a barium enema exam, resulting in a patient fall and a claim against the facility.

The previous examples demonstrate that user errors are a serious problem and should at least be tracked within the facility. As with SMDA and product recall, the appropriate documentation of policies and procedures, education, evaluation, and corrective actions for user errors must be implemented.

## CONCLUSION

The most pressing concern is the need to heighten awareness of both the SMDA and product recall processes in the profession. Policies and procedures must be implemented and used aggressively to reduce the risk of injury, illness, or death of the patients we serve.

To meet this challenge, the medical imaging professional must accept the following guidelines:

1. Demonstrate responsibility to stay current in knowledge and skills for use of equipment and products and for the need for safety in all procedures.
2. Share in knowledge of the profession as mandated by the ASRT Code of Ethics.
3. Be a more informed consumer of medical devices and products by gathering information related to the safety features of all devices and products, rather than depending on the advice of the sales representative.

4. Follow all manufacturers' recommendations for product use, which should include recommendations for a preventive maintenance program.

In other words, the medical imaging professional must accept responsibility for all aspects of patient care.

## NOTES

1. Public Law 101-629 (1990).
2. *ECRI Advisory* (August 1993). ECRI is an independent nonprofit agency established in 1955 and chartered in the state of Pennsylvania. It is widely recognized as the world's leading independent organization committed to improving the safety, efficacy, and cost effectiveness of health care technology.
   ECRI (originally the Emergency Care Research Institute) provides information, evaluation, and consultation to thousands of hospitals, health care organizations, government and planning agencies, voluntary sector organizations, associations, and accrediting agencies worldwide. From the report of the Safe Medical Devices Act of 1990 Conference, presented by Margaret M. deMarteleire, Senior Legal Specialist, ECRI (April 1994).
3. *ECRI Advisory* (April 1994).
4. FDA, *USER Facility Reporting* 5 (Summer 1993).
5. Ibid.
6. FDA, *USER Facility Reporting* 3 (Winter 1992), 1.
7. *Courier Journal/Louisville Times*, 15 October 1988.
8. Marla Poteet, "Latex Reactions Spawn Many New Products," *RS Wavelength* 3, no. 6 (March 1992), 3.
9. "A Computer Glitch Turns Miracle Machine into Monster for Three Cancer Patients," *People*, 24 November 1986.
10. "STAT. MRI Death Leads to Caution. . . . ," *RS Wavelength* 4, no. 9 (June 1993), 23.
11. *Radiology & Imaging Letter*, 1 September 1994, 116.
12. Ibid.
13. Ibid.
14. Ibid.
15. Ibid.
16. *Radiology & Imaging Letter*, 15 May 1994.
17. Ibid.
18. *Radiology & Imaging Letter*, 15 June 1994.
19. Ibid.
20. *FDA Medical Bulletin* 24, no. 1 (May 1994): 6.
21. Ibid.
22. "MR. . . . . SUN," *SIGNA® Users' Newsletter* 9, no. 2 (June 1993).
23. "NIOSH Report on Back Belts Says They Don't Help, May Even Harm," *OSHA Compliance ADVISOR*, 8 August 1994, p. 11.
24. *Biomedical Safety & Standards*, Sample Issue 10 (Brea, GA: Quest Publishing Company, 1994). See *Biomedical Safety & Standards*, 1 February 1992, p. 9.

# 13

# Whistleblower Protection

Ruby D. Fenton

Once there was a concept referred to as "employment at-will." Under that concept, employers and employees were free to sever their employment relationship at will, with or without cause and with or without notice. Over time, that concept has eroded until, as it stands today, it is riddled with exceptions. Both employers and employees are wise to keep up with the current form.

At-will employment is not dead. It is, however, fragile. Today it is illegal for employers to terminate employees under myriad concepts. One such concept is the "whistleblower" exception to the aforementioned employment-at-will doctrine. This exception protects certain classes of employees, who bring to light some form of workplace danger, irresponsibility, or breach of public trust, from being fired. Protection for these employees takes two basic forms: statutory protections (legislative enactments) and common law (laws crafted by the courts under the notion of equity and fair play). This chapter will outline both forms of protection and advise the reader of the types of activities that are protected.

## STATUTORY PROTECTIONS

Presently there exist both state and federal statutes that protect employees who undertake to disclose workplace issues that could harm the public. In addition, the U.S. Constitution protection of free speech may also provide an individual with a cause of action. These statutes are narrowly drawn, having their own scope, procedures, and remedies, and the reader is cautioned to read carefully before assuming that any form of protection exists for him or her.

## First Amendment

The First Amendment to the U.S. Constitution[1] provides that "Congress shall make no law . . . abridging the freedom of speech." The policy underlying this amendment is one that promotes the free exchange of thoughts and ideas among the peoples of this country. However, protection under this and most amendments to the Constitution generally exists only for public sector employees. In other words, employees other than those working for government agencies or companies receiving substantial government funding are probably not covered under this concept of free speech.

Qualified employees are protected under the First Amendment from retaliation by their employers when they "express matters of public concern in a nondisruptive manner."[2] In the case of *Pickering v. Board of Education,* a teacher who had publicly criticized certain of the school board's fiscal policies was protected. Essential to granting protection were the Supreme Court's findings that the matter referred to by the teacher was actually something that concerned the public, and not just a personal concern, and that the manner in which the criticism occurred was not "disruptive." In other decisions, the Supreme Court has declined protection by finding that the expressions were likely to jeopardize discipline or harmony and / or be disruptive to the employer's operations.[3]

## Federal Statutory Protections (Public Sector Employees Only)

There are three major federal statutes which, once again, protect only public employees. Each of these is specifically tailored, and its application is therefore limited.

### The Civil Service Reform Act of 1978[4]

This act covers only federal employees. The act specifically protects disclosures regarding improper activities, including

- Violations of the law
- Gross waste of public funds
- Abuses of governmental authority

This act does not give an employee a cause of action in a court of law. Rather, it provides for a Merit System Protection Board which has the authority to discipline government officials who retaliate against whistleblowers. To prevail, a complaining employee must first show that the behavior complained of fits one of the above categories. Then the employee must provide proof that the official who retaliated against him or her had actual or constructive knowledge that that particular employee had made the subject disclosure. If successful, the employee is entitled to reinstatement (if he or she was terminated by the official), and the official is subject to a range of discipline up to and including termination from the federal civil service for up to five years. Significantly, a prevailing employee may also recover attorney's fees, which clearly provides an incentive for employee representation and strengthens the protections of the act.

### The Whistleblower Protection Act of 1989[5]

This act was passed in an effort to strengthen the Civil Service Reform Act. Under this act, the standard of proof is slightly relaxed, and employees will prevail if they can show that they held a "reasonable belief" that evidence existed of a violation of any law, rule, or regulation; gross mismanagement; gross waste of funds; abuse of authority; or a substantial and specific danger to public health or safety. The revisions set out specific deadlines for both the filing and processing of complaints, which had been absent from the earlier act. Moreover, identity of whistleblowers is expressly proscribed for the time their cases are pending, and the act specifically provides for protective orders for employees throughout the investigatory process. Another important change brought about by this act was a significant shift in the burden of proof. Under this newer act, once it is determined that the whistleblowing activity was a "contributing factor" in whatever personnel action was taken against the whistleblower, corrective action is automatically ordered unless and until the agency can demonstrate, by clear and convincing evidence, that the action would have been taken even if the disclosure had not occurred. The remedies were amended to include provision for civil money penalties not to exceed $1,000.

### Department of Defense Authorization Act[6]

Again, this act was enacted to expand the original protections of the Civil Service Reform Act. This time the amendment expanded the group of employees protected to include employees working on military bases for the Department of Defense. These employees had previously been excluded on the basis of their military status. This amendment extends the protections set forth above, to disclosures to members of Congress or the inspector general of various military departments.

## Federal Statutory Protection (Private Employees)

In addition to the statutes outlined above, Congress has enacted statutes designed to protect employees working in various industries in the private sector.

## The Energy Reorganization Act[7]

This act protects whistleblowers who are licensed by the Nuclear Regulatory Commission, those who have applied for a license, or contractors or subcontractors of an NRC licensee or applicant.

The act protects employees who commence or participate in any way in any proceeding under the Energy Act or the Atomic Energy Act of 1954.[8] Claims generally protected are those relating to the health or safety of employees who work in or around nuclear energy facilities. As with the other acts discussed earlier, employees are not provided a cause of action in a court of law and must commence the complaint procedure by filing with the secretary of labor. The challenged employer can defeat the claim only by producing evidence that the action complained of would have occurred in the absence of the whistleblowing activity.

Unlike acts that protect only federal employees, this act provides equitable and compensatory damages. In other words, prevailing employees are entitled to reinstatement and back pay (as with the other acts) but may also qualify for compensatory damages for embarrassment and humiliation, as well as attorney's fees.

## The Federal Mine Safety and Health Act[9]

This act provides protection for mineworkers who disclose safety hazards in their working conditions. Under this act, employees may demand inspections and may be allowed to refuse to work under conditions that could cause long- or short-term health consequences.

## Occupational Safety and Health Act (OSHA)[10]

This act protects private employees working in a wide variety of industries. Employees are protected from retaliation by their employers when requesting inspections based on a belief that some safety violation threatens physical harm or presents an imminent danger of physical harm. Like the act protecting mineworkers, this act allows work refusal under certain circumstances.

## Antiretaliation Protections Under Other Federal Acts

Congress has passed a number of acts that prohibit discrimination in employment and/or set minimum standards for terms and conditions of covered employment.[11] In addition to those primary protections are what are generally referred to as antiretaliation provisions. Those provisions preclude any form of adverse employment action against an employee exercising rights under the underlying act. For example, Title VII, or the Civil Rights Act, is designed to protect employees from discrimination in the terms and conditions of their jobs on the basis of race, sex, religion, and so on.[12] The Equal Employment Opportunity Commission (EEOC) was established under that same act for the purpose of investigating, and conciliating where possible, claims raised under the act. At the same time, Congress included protection for individuals who filed suit under this act from being retaliated against by their employers, when that retaliation is based on the fact that an employee is exercising his or her statutory rights. The antiretaliation provision also protects fellow employees and others who are called upon to provide information or testimony in the course of investigating the claim of discrimination.

There are many other such acts with effectively identical provisions. These include the Age Discrimination in Employment Act,[13] the Americans with Disabilities Act,[14] the Equal Pay Act,[15] and the National Labor Relations Act.[16] It is important to note that, under the antiretaliation provisions of these and of most acts, it is not necessary that an employee prevail on his or her underlying claim (for instance, that a work hazard exists or that they have been discriminated against because of their age) in order to be protected against retaliation. Those provisions apply whether or not the employee ultimately prevails in proving the claim. In other words, the claim of retaliation under these acts is separate and distinct from the claim raised under the substantive provisions of the act. In fact, claims of retaliation are often easier to win than those advanced initially. Employees are cautioned, however, that, to win a retaliation claim, they must prove that some form of adverse employment consequences have been suffered as a direct result of engaging in the protected activity of seeking relief provided by one or more of these acts, and not all negative acts on the part of an employer will constitute a violation of the antiretaliation provisions. Stated another way, it is a common misconception among those who have claimed workplace discrimination that they are then insulated from any and all adverse actions taken by their employer from the date of their claim forward. This just isn't true. If poor performance or insubordination warrant discipline or discharge, and such action would be taken in the normal course of business absent the charge of discrimination, the employer will be relieved of liability for retaliation.

## State Statutory Protection (Government Employees)

As of this writing, 24 states have statutes that protect government-employed whistleblowers. The protections afforded these employees parallel those provided by federal statutes protecting federal employees, as previously discussed. These states are Alaska, Arizona, California, Colorado, Delaware, Florida, Illinois, Indiana, Iowa, Kansas, Kentucky, Maryland, Missouri, North Carolina, Oklahoma, Oregon, Pennsylvania, South

Carolina, Tennessee, Texas, Utah, Washington, West Virginia, and Wisconsin.[17] The protections for these employees are generally found in the statutes establishing terms and conditions of government, or merit system employees. Generally speaking, government employees are not at-will employees and may be discharged only for cause. In addition to that protection, these employees are generally provided protection for policing their employing agencies when that activity takes the form of disclosing some form of workplace danger, irresponsibility, or breach of public trust, including violations of the law, waste of public funds, and abuses of governmental authority. These acts generally contain some form of the following limitations:

- The complaint must be made in good faith.
- The employee may not refuse to work unless there exists an imminent and substantial danger of death or serious injury.
- The employee may not disclose to the public confidential information of the agency.

Remedies include reinstatement of the whistleblower's position and the imposition of penalties on employers, which may include reprimands, imprisonment, or monetary fines. California and Alaska allow recovery for punitive damages, and North Carolina allows treble damages for whistleblower violations.

## COMMON LAW PROTECTION FOR WHISTLEBLOWERS

In addition to the legislatively created exceptions to the employment-at-will doctrine are those crafted by both state and federal courts. In almost every state there now exists a cause of action for wrongful discharge. Under this theory, an employer may not discharge an employee who would otherwise be considered at-will, if the discharge would violate some form of established public policy. The earliest examples of cases filed under this theory are those in which an employee was discharged because he or she had pursued their rights under their state's worker's compensation laws. In creating the cause of action for wrongful discharge, courts reasoned that it was not appropriate for an employer to discharge an employee simply because that employee had exercised a right given that employee by the legislature.

The concept of wrongful discharge for violation of public policy later expanded, and courts refined the standards necessary for bringing a claim under this theory. As it now stands, in order to prevail, an employee must show that he or she was discharged either for exercising a right given him or her by statute or for refusing to violate a law when asked to do so by the employer. In addition, courts will recognize a cause of action for wrongful discharge when an employee can prove that he or she was discharged for reporting unlawful employer conduct to an investigative or regulatory agency. The conduct for which the employee is terminated, however, must advance the public policy relied upon in order to state a claim for wrongful discharge. For example, one such case was dismissed because the court determined that the banking violations the employee had reported posed no serious threat to the health and safety of the citizens of the state.[18]

Jurisdictions recognizing the public policy exception to the employment-at-will doctrine as of this writing include all states with the exception of Delaware, Florida, Georgia, Louisiana, and New York. States where there is no clear expression of intent to allow or disallow the exception are Maine and Rhode Island.

When an employee wins a claim of wrongful discharge, most jurisdictions will award compensatory and even punitive damages when the employer's conduct is sufficiently outrageous. Wisconsin, however, limits recovery to reinstatement with back pay.

## CONCLUSION

Whistleblowing is indeed protected under a variety of legal theories. These theories are, however, diverse and command a fairly high standard of proof. Moreover, not all employees are covered in all situations. As a result, when and if an employee is confronted with a perceived violation of public trust or a potential violation of the law on the part of his or her employer, that employee should consult legal counsel to determine what, if any, protection is available upon disclosure of the problem. Generally, courts embrace the opportunity to right these wrongs and encourage conscientious disclosures on the part of employees as a way of ensuring employer compliance with the law and promoting consumer protection. However, the practical ramifications of choosing to disclose such activity should also be taken into account. Notwithstanding the express legal protections, life can still be difficult for an employee who chooses such a path. For that reason, equally encouraged by the courts—indeed required by some jurisdictions—it is recommended by this author that all internal procedures for remedying the kinds of situations outlined in this chapter be examined and utilized where they will be effective. As with any other kind of claim, a lawsuit is never the fastest and almost never the most effective method for resolving workplace issues. On the other hand, that route is available under the circumstances set out above and when there exist no other alternatives.

# NOTES

1. "Congress shall make no law respecting an establishment of religion, or prohibiting the free exercise thereof; or abridging the freedom of speech, or of the press; or the rights of the people to peaceably assemble, and to petition the Government for redress of grievances." Amendment I, *Constitution of the United States,* ratified 1791.
2. Pickering v. Board of Education, 391 U.S. 563 (1968).
3. Rankin v. McPherson, 483 U.S. 378 (1987).
4. 5 U.S.C. §2301 et seq.
5. 5 U.S.C. §1201 et seq.
6. 10 U.S.C. §1587 et seq.
7. 41 U.S.C. §5801–5891.
8. 42 U.S.C. §2011 et seq.
9. 30 U.S.C. §815 et seq.
10. 29 U.S.C. §657 et seq.
11. Age Discrimination in Employment Act, 29 U.S.C. §621 et seq.; The Clean Air Act, 42 U.S.C. §7401 et seq.; Employee Retirement Income Security Act, 29 U.S.C. §1001 et seq.
12. Equal Employment Opportunity Act ("Civil Rights Act"), 42 U.S.C. §2000e et seq., as amended by the Civil Rights Act of 1991; Fair Labor Standards Act, 29 U.S.C. §215(a)(3)(1988).
13. Age Discrimination in Employment Act, 29 U.S.C. §621 et seq.
14. Americans with Disabilities Act, 42 U.S.C. §12101 et seq.
15. Equal Pay Act, 29 U.S.C. §206(d).
16. National Labor Relations Act, 29 U.S.C. §151 et seq.
17. Alaska Stat. Section 39.90.100 et seq. (1991 Supp.).
    Ariz. Rev. Stat. Ann. Section 38-531 et seq. (West Supp. 1991).
    Cal. Government Code Section 10540 et seq. (West Supp. 1992).
    Colo. Rev. Stat. Section 24-50.5-101 et seq. (West 1990).
    Del. Code Ann. tit. 29, Section 5115 (1991).
    Fla. Stat. Ann. Section 112.3187 (West Supp. 1992).
    Ill. Ann. Stat. Ch. 127, Paragraph 63b119c.1 (Smith-Hurd Supp. 1991).
    Ind. Code Ann. Section 4-15-10-4 (Burns 1990).
    Iowa Code Ann. Section 79.28 et seq. (West 1991).
    Kan. Stat. Ann. Section 75-2973 (1991 Supp.).
    Ky. Rev. Stat. Ann. Section 61-101 et seq. (1986).
    Maryland Ann. Code art. 64A Section 12F et seq. (1991 Supp.).
    Mo. Rev. Stat. Section 105.055 (Vernon Supp. 1992).
    N.C. Gen. Stat. Section 126-84 et seq. (1991).
    Okla. Stat. tit. 74, Section 841.7 et seq. (West 1987 & 1992 Supp.).
    Or. Rev. Stat. Section 659.505 et seq. (1991).
    43 Pa. Cons. Stat. Section 1421 et seq. (Purdon 1991).
    S.C. Code Ann. Section 8-27-et seq. (Law. Co-op. Supp. 1991).
    Tenn. Code Ann. Section 49-50-1401 et seq. (1990).
    Tex. Rev. Civ. Stat. Ann. art. 6252-16a (Vernon Supp. 1992).
    Utah Code Ann. Section 67-21-1 et seq. (1986 & 1991 Supp.).
    Wash. Rev. Code Ann. Section 42.40.010 et seq. (1990).
    W. Va. Code Section 6C-1-1 et seq. (1990).
    Wis. Stat. Ann. Section 230.80 et seq. (West 1987 & 1991 Supp.).
18. Hicks v. Resolution Trust Corp., 736 F. Supp. 812 (N.D. Ill. 1990).

# C H A P T E R
# 14

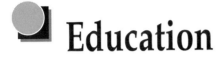

# Education

Ann M. Obergfell

**A** recurring theme throughout the review of legal and ethical issues affecting the practices of diagnostic imaging and therapeutic radiology is the concept of education. A review of educational requirements for professionals with an analysis of methods used for assessing and evaluating competency is imperative when preparing to meet the changing needs of the health care consumer. Likewise, keeping current with the depth and breadth of knowledge is the obligation of all radiologic science professionals. The new patient consumer has greater expectations of those who provide services and require that these professionals offer enough information that an educated and informed consent to services may be rendered. Therefore, patient education must be a part of every radiologic science professional's clinical practice.

The skill of individuals working in the radiologic science professions is contingent upon pre-professional, professional, and continuing education.

## PRE-PROFESSIONAL EDUCATION

Programs in radiography, radiation therapy, nuclear medicine, and sonography have a variety of pre-professional requirements that range from high school diploma or GED to variable college general education requirements. Regardless of the program requirements, as the profession advances and changes, so must the preparation level of those entering the disciplines. While it has always been recommended that pre-professional students be prepared in math and the sciences, it will be even more important as they meet the challenges of the ever-expanding technological professions. Any person entering the radiologic sciences must have in-depth knowledge of anatomical structure and function. Computed tomography, magnetic resonance imaging, sonography, and cardiovascular interventional radiography require a keen understanding of very specific physiological and anatomical principles.

As health care changes and patient's rights become more readily recognized, health care professionals will be required to have excellent communication skills and be able to deal with the emotional needs of severely sick and injured people. Pre-professionals with courses in communication, interpersonal relationships, and psychology will be better prepared to understand the patient care and ethical concerns of the patient and the discipline.

The written word is as important as the spoken one and individuals entering these professions must be able to express themselves effectively in writing. Courses in English composition or business writing will be valuable to the pre-professional student.

Computerized equipment in imaging and therapy departments is no longer the exception but the norm. Therefore, anyone interested in entering the radiologic sciences must be computer literate.

A sample pre-professional curriculum that could be adopted by all programs might include:

- English composition
- Mathematics
- Chemistry
- Physics
- Communication
- Anatomy and physiology
- Computer applications
- Psychology

It has become clear to anyone who understands and works closely with radiologic science professionals that the complexities of the technological environment require that individuals entering the professions be both academically and experientially prepared to meet the challenges of the curriculum and the practice. Programs may want to consider requiring an observation or volunteer period in a diagnostic imaging facility for all pre-professional candidates.

## PROFESSIONAL

The professional curricula for radiography, nuclear medicine, radiation therapy, and sonography must continually adjust to the rapidly changing technology. As new technologies enter the imaging and therapy fields, the curricula are updated to include the theory as well as the practical application. An accredited educational program must develop program curriculum which meet the requirements established in the specific discipline's educational standards as well as meeting the needs of the discipline and the community which it serves.

The following content areas are just a sampling of the minimum educational standards established for educational programs in radiography, nuclear medicine, radiation therapy, and diagnostic medical sonography:[1]

### Content areas recognized in all programs standards

| | |
|---|---|
| medical ethics and law | quality assurance |
| patient care | computer literacy |
| medical terminology | clinical education |
| human structure and function | pathology |

### Radiography, nuclear medicine, radiation therapy

radiation biology
radiation safety
radiation physics

### Radiography

radiographic procedures
principles of radiographic exposures
imaging equipment
film processing
evaluation of radiographs

### Nuclear medicine

nuclear instrumentation
statistics
radionuclide chemistry and radiopharmacy
in-vivo and in-vitro procedures
radionuclide therapy

### Radiation oncology

radiation oncology
oncologic pathology
radiation oncology technique
clinical dosimetry
introduction to hyperthermia

### Diagnostic medical sonography

human physiology and hemodynamics
sectional sonographic anatomy
permanent image record critique
ultrasound instrumentation
acoustical physics
doppler ultrasound principles
medical ultrasound
cardiac and circulatory physiology
pathophysiology
cardiac sonography procedures

While these minimum guidelines are subject to change each time the educational standards are revised and updated, program faculty must utilize these guidelines when setting up program curricula and continue to make changes as part of an ongoing evaluation of the effectiveness of the program.

Additional educational opportunities in administration, management, and education may be required as the radiologic sciences expand and as health care changes to meet the diverse needs of society. Many facilities require advanced degrees in business for supervisory or management positions. Education courses will be beneficial as the role of the professional expands in the areas of patient education, clinical supervision, and mentoring programs.

Imaging and therapy department administrators should utilize the professional educational requirements when determining criterion referenced job descriptions and employment expectations for current and future positions. Special or additional educational requirements should be employed when defining positions which utilize special skills such as education, supervision, advanced imaging, and quality assurance.

## PROFESSIONAL COMPETENCY

Changes in health care accreditation standards and the litigious nature of society have forced health care facilities to evaluate the competencies of all employees. These evaluations range from written examinations to clinical skill testing and are completed on either a formal or informal basis.

Facilities should develop a system of competency evaluation that begins at the time of employment and continues at least annually throughout the employment period. Competency evaluation should include all members of the team from the medical staff to the physical plant crew members. Ensuring quality health care service is the responsibility of everyone in the facility and therefore the competency of each employee and provider must be reviewed. A system that integrates job descriptions, continuing education, and competency evaluation best serves the facility and the patients.

## Criterion Referenced Job Descriptions

The administration of the facility, with input from employees, should establish criterion referenced job descriptions for each position in the facility. This not only directs employment duties but assures that all aspects of the delivery of services are covered by a specific position or combination of positions.

After position descriptions are developed, a task list must be formulated. The facility can use these lists to establish the essential functions of each position; the lists can be distributed to applicants and posted on job boards. The essential functions assist the potential applicant in understanding the requirements of the position. The task list can also be used to create checklists for evaluation purposes.

Once an individual is employed by the facility, the checklist and criterion referenced job description can be used to direct the orientation process, the probationary period, and the remainder of the employment term. In-service programs, such as infection control, new equipment and procedure orientation, and facility safety, can be presented to employees based on the specific proficiency. These sessions can be followed by clinical practice and competency evaluation.

## PROFESSIONAL EDUCATION

Professional continuing education generally takes two forms: (1) educational meetings or seminars away from the employment setting and (2) in-service sessions designed to meet the needs of the facility. There are a number of mechanisms available for continuing professional education and it is up the individual to decide what method best meets his or her needs. A combination of several methods, such as attending professional meetings, participating in facility in-service, reading professional journals, and attending courses in related or complimentary fields, will give the professional a better understanding of what is current and important to the radiologic sciences.

## Continuing Education

The most common form of professional continuing education is the educational seminars offered by national, state, and local professional organizations. These organizations offer a variety of educational opportunities ranging from several-day annual meetings to one-day seminars on a specific topic, such as mammography or advanced imaging modalities. The business of the profession is usually part of these sessions and it is important that the radiologic science professional be familiar not only with the technological advances of the discipline but with the political and societal pressures, which affect the delivery of care and the advancement of the profession.

Most professional organizations have journals available to the membership. These journals are generally peer reviewed and offer the reader timely topics affecting or changing the way care should be delivered. Most hospital libraries have subscriptions to these journals; if they do not, departmental administration should request that they be included in the periodicals available for all facility personnel. Smaller facilities may wish to order journals to be kept in a lounge or quiet area in the building easily accessible to office or clinic personnel. Articles available in these journals are often used to establish the standard of care expected of a professional. Therefore, it is imperative that each professional read the journals which relate to the individual's area of expertise.

Another mechanism for receiving professional continuing education is through private for-profit continuing education businesses, which offer educational programs in the radiologic sciences. Some of these businesses are national in scope, while others are more regional in nature. In either case, they offer  viable educational opportunities for members of the radiologic sciences.

## In-Service Education

Traditionally, in-service programs in imaging departments have been haphazard attempts to meet the individual department's educational needs. The advent of mandatory continuing education, and the expanding role of the technologist and therapist, requires a change in the approach to in-service education. Facility education coordinators usually prepare nursing education programs and are unfamiliar with the needs of radiologic science professionals. Therefore, either administrative directors of imaging and therapy departments must work with the education department to prepare and implement programs for employees or an education position should be developed within the department to prepare, coordinate, and organize quality educational programs.

In-services should be planned in advance so that the presentations can be well prepared and approved for continuing education credit. At least twelve sessions per year (one per month) should be offered. The programs should be approved by the state, where applicable, or by a recognized continuing education evaluation mechanism (RCEEM) such as the American Society of Radiologic Technologists (ASRT). Approval by the American Medical Association (AMA) and the American Nursing Association (ANA) is acceptable as long as the topics approved are relevant to the radiologic sciences.

Programs should be developed around the criterion referenced job descriptions and the policies and procedures established for the facility. For example, if competency in Cardiopulmonary resuscitation (CPR) is required in the job description, than CPR should be included in the educational program established for the facility or, if the department has a policy that permits technologists to perform venipuncture and requires regular updates on contrast media, the facility should include such programs in the educational plan.

Facility educational coordinators should plan innovative programs utilizing the plethora of available sources in any health care setting. Pharmaceutical representatives can offer programs on the latest contrast, radiopharmaceutical, or other related medication; equipment application specialists can prepare and present sessions on new technologies; nurses can provide sessions on patient care skills; infection control personnel can discuss current trends in the prevention of disease transmission; risk management and safety personnel can offer sessions on hospital procedures and guidelines; physicians can offer sessions on their particular area of expertise; and technologists and therapists can present the newest modalities or innovations in the field. The design and topics of educational programming are only limited by the imagination of the persons planning the sessions.

Health care facilities may utilize the job description as part of a needs assessment when determining the type and scope of educational in-service programs. Traditional lecture presentations are of great value but there are many other useful methods of organizing educational opportunities. Staff technologists can present mini-sessions on new technologies or prepare refresher courses on seldom-used or problem procedures. Brainstorming discussion methods can help resolve problem issues in the department or clinic. Case studies can be presented and problem solving techniques can be incorporated as part of the continuing education and quality assurance program.

A review of department policies and procedures can be offered at the monthly in-service session or at regularly scheduled staff meetings. This process assures that all employees are familiar with the policies of the facility, and will help flush out policies that are outdated or do not meet the needs of the facility or the standard of the community.

Good quality educational opportunities for all employees assists the facility to reach its goal of providing quality competent care to the patient consumer and to meet accreditation and regulatory standards.

Ensuring that all employees remain current in their respective fields is an important obligation of all employers. The current trends of cross training and patient centered care can be accomplished through a well planned continuing education or in-service program. Departmental administration should work with the staff to develop a program that meets the needs of the staff and the facility.

## Related College Courses

Many communities have vocational schools, colleges, or universities that offer courses to non-traditional students. Courses in computers, supervision, education, and interpersonal relationships are offered in the evening, on weekends, as short courses, and at off-campus locations to meet the needs of full-time employees.

Some employers offer tuition remission programs, which allow employees to be reimbursed for the cost of courses related to the employment. Others contract with the local educational institution to offer courses for a group of employees at a discounted rate or at the employment facility.

All continuing education opportunities benefit not only the individual but the facility and the profession. The employee will be better able to handle the changing demands of the health care delivery system, the facility will have competent employees who are current in their field and are able to provide quality patient care, and the profession will receive greater credibility with a better educated membership.

## Competency Evaluation

A system of evaluation should be developed, implemented, and reviewed by the facility to ensure that each employee is meeting the expectations outlined in the job description and facility goals.

Once the specific competencies required for the position are established, methods of evaluation must be developed. Each competency should be analyzed to determine the best method of evaluation: oral or written examination in the cognitive domain, demonstration of skill in the psychomotor domain, behavioral evaluation in the affective domain, or through some combination of the three.

Level of competency must be determined for each skill. This is determined by the value placed on the skill by the facility. For some skills, a 75% rating may be required, but if the competency is one in which accuracy and competency are paramount then a rating closer to 100% may be placed on the skill (for example, identifying the appropriate patient is a skill that requires 100% accuracy). A 100% accuracy level is a difficult standard; a level of perhaps 95–98 may be more realistic on some critical tasks.

Reviewing employee competence by assessing cognitive, psychomotor, and affective behaviors should be completed at least annually. Ignoring evaluation because an employee has reached a certain level only serves to encourage a stagnant and potentially mediocre work environment because the employee feels no obligation to maintain competency or to improve skills and knowledge.

## Cognitive Evaluation

Professionals are not only required to be competent on specific behaviors, they must also have up-to-date knowledge of information such as safety procedures, OSHA guidelines, blood-borne and airborne pathogen requirements, medical terminology, and department policies. Facilities can select a team of professionals who will work together to create objectives for each area deemed important for employee competency. In-service programs can be presented based on the identified objectives.

Knowledge gained and retained by the employee may be measured through the use of written evaluation (i.e., quiz or test). The exams may be given at intervals throughout the employment period. Medical terminology and abbreviation tests may be given annually, while a quiz on infection control policies may be given immediately following a regularly scheduled in-service and again in three months to see if the information is being retained.

Any time a department policy or procedure is added or changed, all employees should be advised of the change and a notice should be posted in an area accessible to all employees. Quizzes on policies can be given throughout the year at regularly scheduled staff meetings or in-services.

## Psychomotor Evaluation

If the competency requires the demonstration of specific skills (e.g., the employee must be able to perform a lumbar spine series or be able to take an accurate blood pressure), then a task list of observable skills for each procedure should be incorporated into a performance evaluation instrument. A supervisor can check the competency of the employee by using the performance evaluation form and observing the procedure.

If the employee is not successful in the competency evaluation, a system of remediation should be implemented. Remediation may include a review of literature on the specific competency or a hands-on review (with a phantom if actual exposure is required, or with a fellow employee if the skill requires a human subject but no radiation exposure).

Departments may develop mentoring programs whereby competent employees who are interested will work with employees who do not successfully complete the evaluation process. The mentor system can also be utilized with new employees or with students who participate in clinical education at the facility. Each employee who is selected or volunteers to mentor must understand the importance of his or her role within the system and must be prepared to meet special challenges that may arise. A successful mentoring program will advance the needs of the facility and the individual employees.

When a competency has been completed successfully, documentation of the competency evaluation can be incorporated in the employee's file and used for performance and promotion reviews.

Facility accreditation and quality assurance programs may require that data on performance evaluation be incorporated in department records. This type of data is generally collected without employee identification and is used to show that the department is meeting the education and evaluation requirements of accreditation. Quality assurance programs may utilize the data to demonstrate trends and to show that the department and its employees are participating in a continual system of assessment and review.

Another important aspect of quality assurance programs that can be used for evaluating performance is through the ongoing system of repeat analysis. If the facility utilizes repeat analysis as part of their quality assurance program and keeps a record not only of the number of errors but the types of errors, a remediation process can be implemented to assist the employees in correcting or perfecting their imaging skills. For example, if it is discovered that an employee must continually repeat oblique lumbar spine projections, then a supervisor, mentor, or educational coordinator can work with the employee to discover the cause and correct the problem. Through a continuing repeat analysis program, the effectiveness of the corrective action can be evaluated.

## Affective Evaluation

Radiologic science professionals must not only be technologically proficient and able to adapt to the ever-changing face of health care delivery, but must exhibit behavior appropriate to the helping professions. Evaluation of these behaviors is often perceived as subjective. However, given specific criteria, the evaluation can be performed in an objective fashion, and is as important to a total competency evaluation system as the perceptually more objective psychomotor and cognitive reviews. An example of assessing affective behavior may include how an employee answers the phone: "Diagnostic imaging, this is Mary Smith, may I help you?" instead of "x-ray, what do you want?"

Areas of evaluation should include a review of interpersonal relationships with patients, peers, administration, and other members of the health care team; ability to work as part of the team; and the ability to behave as expected in the Code of Ethics[2] and the Patient's Bill of Rights.[3] These types of behaviors all involve the affective domain.

The nature of affective evaluation requires that a system use several methods of review, including performance observation, self evaluation, patient questionnaires, and peer review. Any evaluation tool utilized by the facility should have specific actions identified and use terms which are measurable.

Individuals in the radiologic sciences are professionals and the nature of the work requires that they interact with a variety of people in a variety of settings. Consideration, thoughtfulness, compassion, caring, and respect are but a few of the traits expected of members of the helping professions. While it is hoped that these characteristics would be inherent in the health care provider, it is clear that many are learned behaviors, and are as critical to the delivery of care as the ability to perform procedures or treatments. Therefore it is imperative that these appropriate behaviors be learned and followed by anyone who is a member of the radiologic sciences. Evaluation reinforces the importance of these traits to the delivery of good quality care.

## Patient Education

The consumer patient is better educated and is gathering information on health care delivery from many sources, including the media, politicians, insurance companies, and other health care watch dogs. The deluge of information bombarding the consumer runs the gamut from accurate to inaccurate, so the health care industry, and in particular radiologic science professionals, must develop a plan for educating the public about the health care system.

Facilities that offer health care services should incorporate patient education into the departmental policies and procedures. Both professional and nonprofessional employees should be able to answer questions asked by patients and should be able to intelligently explain what will be happening before, during, and after a procedure or treatment.

Larger facilities may employ or develop a position of patient educator to handle all scheduling and patient education for the department. The patient educator can schedule and explain procedures; offer inservices for physicians who order procedures for patients at the facility and for nursing floor personnel who are responsible for prepping in-patients; develop patient education brochures or videotapes explaining procedures and protocols; and visit in-patients prior to the scheduled procedure to answer questions.

Small clinics or offices may include patient education in the criterion referenced job description of any employee who works closely with patients. Office staff, including the physician, should work together to develop a system whereby any patient entering the facility can have their questions answered in a timely and accurate manner.

Educated patients are generally more cooperative, able to make decisions concerning their care, and are better able to follow pre- and post-procedural and treatment protocol.

## CONCLUSION

Pre-professional, professional, and continuing education play important roles in the development of the radiologic science professional. Practitioners must not only have the fundamental knowledge necessary to practice, but must be able to adapt easily to the ever-changing technology without losing sight of the needs of the patient.

Educational opportunities abound, and it is the responsibility of the professional to keep abreast of new trends in technology, changes in standards, and issues affecting the practice and the profession. Professional organizations, private businesses, and health care facilities all offer educational programs and in-services.

Accreditation standards and health care reform require that the knowledge and skill level of health professionals be evaluated on a regular basis. Competency evaluation is used to not only to evaluate individual skill but to assist in creating a more cohesive and quality department, clinic, or office. Weaknesses in the staff and system can be identified; remediation programs can be developed, implemented, and reviewed; and strengths can be rewarded.

The patient consumer's expectations are great and it is important that the radiologic science professional take an active role in educationing the patient about diagnostic or therapeutic procedures. Administration and staff should work together to create a professional environment that is conducive to quality service and professional growth.

## N O T E S

1. Essentials and Guidelines of an Accredited Educational Program for the Radiographer., Adopted by the Joint Review Committee on Education in Radiologic Technology, Chicago, IL, 1994.

   Essentials and Guidelines of an Accredited Educational Program for the Diagnostic Medical Sonographer, 1987.

   Essentials and Guidelines of an Accredited Educational Program for the Radiation Therapist, 1994.

   Essentials and Guidelines for an Accredited Educational Program for the Nuclear Medicine Technologist, Adopted by the Joint Review Committee on Education in Nuclear Medicine Technology, Salt Lake City, UT, 1991.
2. Code of Ethics for Radiologic Technologists, adopted by American Society of Radiologic Technologists and the American Registry of Radiologic Technologists. Revised 1994.
3. Patient's Bill of Rights, American Hospital Association, 1992.

# Code of Ethics

1. The Radiologic Technologist conducts himself/ herself in a professional manner, responds to patient needs and supports colleagues and associates in providing quality patient care.

2. The Radiologic Technologist acts to advance the principle objective of the profession to provide services to humanity with full respect for the dignity of mankind.

3. The Radiologic Technologist delivers patient care and service unrestricted by concerns of personal attributes or the nature of the disease or illness, and without discrimination, regardless of sex, race, creed, religion, or socioeconomic status.

4. The Radiologic Technologist practices technology founded upon theoretical knowledge and concepts, utilizes equipment and accessories consistent with purpose for which it has been designed, and employs procedures and techniques appropriately.

5. The Radiologic Technologist assesses situations, exercises care, discretion and judgment, assumes responsibility for professional decisions, and acts in the best interest of the patient.

6. The Radiologic Technologist acts as an agent through observation and communication to obtain pertinent information of the physician to aid in the diagnosis and treatment management of the patient, and recognizes that interpretation and diagnosis are outside the scope of practice for the profession.

7. The Radiologic Technologist utilizes equipment and accessories, employs techniques and procedures, performs services in accordance with an accepted standard of practice, and demonstrates expertise in minimizing the radiation exposure to the patient, self and other members of the health care team.

8. The Radiologic Technologist practices ethical conduct appropriate to the profession, and protects the patient's right to quality radiologic technology care.

9. The Radiologic Technologist respects confidences entrusted in the course of professional practice, respects the patient's right to privacy, and reveals confidential information only as required by law or to protect the welfare of the individuals or the community.

10. The Radiologic Technologist continually strives to improve knowledge and skills by participating in educational and professional activities, sharing knowledge with colleagues and investigating new and innovative aspects of professional practice. One means available to improve knowledge and skills is through professional continuing education.

Adopted by: The American Society of Radiologic Technologists
The American Registry of Radiologic Technologists

Rev. 7/94

## Canadian Association of
## Medical Radiation Technologists

# Code of Ethics

The Canadian Association of Medical Radiation Technologists recognizes its obligation to identify and promote professional standards of conduct and performance. The execution of such standards is the personal responsibility of each member.

The Code of Ethics requires that every member shall:

- provide service with dignity and respect to all people regardless of race, national or ethnic origin, colour, sex, religion, age, type of illness, mental or physical challenges;
- encourage the trust and confidence of the public through high standards of professional competence, conduct, and appearance;
- conduct all technical procedures with due regard to current radiation safety standards;
- practise only those procedures for which the necessary qualifications are held unless such procedures have been properly delegated by an appropriate medical authority and for which the technologist has received adequate training to an acceptable level of competence;
- practise only those disciplines of medical radiation technology for which he or she has been certified by the C.A.M.R.T. and is currently competent;
- be mindful that patients must seek diagnostic information from their treating physician. In those instances where a discreet comment to the appropriate authority may assist diagnosis or treatment, the technologist may feel morally obliged to provide one;
- preserve and protect the confidentiality of any information, either medical or personal, acquired through professional contact with the patient. An exception may be appropriate when the disclosure of such information is necessary to the treatment of the patient, the safety of other patients or health care providers, or is a legal requirement;
- cooperate with other health care providers;
- advance the art and science of medical radiation technology through ongoing professional development; and
- recognize the participation and support of our association is a professional responsibility.

June 1991

## Management Advisory

## Patient and Community Relations

# A Patient's Bill of Rights

## Introduction

Effective health care requires collaboration between patients and physicians and other health care professionals. Open and honest communication, respect for personal and professional values, and sensitivity to differences are integral to optimal patient care. As the setting for the provision of health services, hospitals must provide a foundation for understanding and respecting the rights and responsibilities of patients, their families, physicians, and other caregivers. Hospitals must ensure a health care ethic that respects the role of patients in decision making about treatment choices and other aspects of their care. Hospitals must be sensitive to cultural, racial, linguistic, religious, age, gender, and other differences as well as the needs of persons with disabilities.

The American Hospital Association presents A Patient's Bill of Rights with the expectation that it will contribute to more effective patient care and be supported by the hospital on behalf of the institution, its medical staff, employees, and patients. The American Hospital Association encourages health care institutions to tailor this bill of rights to their patient community by translating and/or simplifying the language of this bill of rights as may be necessary to ensure that patients and their families understand their rights and responsibilities.

## Bill of Rights*

1. The patient has the right to considerate and respectful care.
2. The patient has the right to and is encouraged to obtain from physicians and other direct caregivers relevant, current, and understandable information concerning diagnosis, treatment, and prognosis.

   Except in emergencies when the patient lacks decision-making capacity and the need for treatment is urgent, the patient is entitled to the opportunity to discuss and request information related to the specific procedures and/ or treatments, the risks involved, the possible length of recuperation, and the medically reasonable alternatives and their accompanying risks and benefits.

   Patients have the right to know the identity of physicians, nurses, and others involved in their care, as well as when those involved are students, residents, or other trainees. The patient also has the right to know the immediate and long-term financial implications of treatment choices, insofar as they are known.
3. The patient has the right to make decisions about the plan of care prior to and during the course of treatment and to refuse a recommended treatment or plan of care to the extent permitted by law and hospital policy and to be informed of the medical consequences of this action. In case of such refusal, the patient is entitled to other appropriate care and services that the hospital provides or transfers to another hospital. The hospital should notify patients of any policy that might affect patient choice within the institution.
4. The patient has the right to have an advance directive (such as a living will, health care proxy, or durable power of attorney for health care) concerning treatment or designating a surrogate decision maker with the expectation that the hospital will honor the intent

   *(continued)*

*These rights can be exercised on the patient's behalf by a designated surrogate or proxy decision maker if the patient lacks decision-making capacity, is legally incompetent, or is a minor.*

# A Patient's Bill of Rights (continued)

of that directive to the extent permitted by law and hospital policy.

Health care institutions must advise patients of their rights under state law and hospital policy to make informed medical choices, ask if the patient has an advance directive, and include that information in patient records. The patient has the right to timely information about hospital policy that may limit its ability to implement fully a legally valid advance directive.

5. The patient has the right to every consideration of privacy. Case discussion, consultation, examination, and treatment should be conducted so as to protect each patient's privacy.

6. The patient has the right to expect that all communications and records pertaining to his/her care will be treated as confidential by the hospital, except in cases such as suspected abuse and public health hazards when reporting is permitted or required by law. The patient has the right to expect that the hospital will emphasize the confidentiality of this information when it releases it to any other parties entitled to review information in these records.

7. The patient has the right to review the records pertaining to his/her medical care and to have the information explained or interpreted as necessary, except when restricted by law.

8. The patient has the right to expect that, within its capacity and policies, a hospital will make reasonable response to the request of a patient for appropriate and medically indicated care and services. The hospital must provide evaluation, service, and/or referral as indicated by the urgency of the case. When medically appropriate and legally permissible, or when a patient has so requested, a patient may be transferred to another facility. The institution to which the patient is to be transferred must first have accepted the patient for transfer. The patient must also have the benefit of complete information and explanation concerning the need for, risks, benefits, and alternatives to such a transfer.

9. The patient has the right to ask and

be informed of the existence of business relationships among the hospital, educational institution, other health care providers, or payers that may influence the patient's treatment and care.

10. The patient has the right to consent to or decline to participate in proposed research studies or human experimentation affecting care and treatment or requiring direct patient involvement, and to have those studies fully explained prior to consent. A patient who declines to participate in research or experimentation is entitled to the most effective care that the hospital can otherwise provide.

11. The patient has the right to expect reasonable continuity of care when appropriate and to be informed by physicians and other caregivers of available and realistic patient care options when hospital care is no longer appropriate.

12. The patient has the right to be informed of hospital policies and practices that relate to patient care, treatment, and responsibilities. The patient has the right to be informed of available resources for resolving disputes, grievances, and conflicts, such as ethics committees, patient representatives, or other mechanisms available in the institution. The patient has the right to be informed of the hospital's charges for services and available payment methods.

The collaborative nature of health care requires that patients, or their families/ surrogates, participate in their care. The effectiveness of care and patient satisfaction with the course of treatment depend, in part, on the patient fulfilling certain responsibilities. Patients are responsible for providing information about past illnesses, hospitalizations, medications, and other matters related to health status. To participate effectively in decision making, patients must be encouraged to take responsibility for requesting additional information or clarification about their health status or treatment when they do not fully understand information and instructions. Patients are also responsible for ensuring that the health care institution has a copy of their written advance directive if they have one. Patients are responsible for informing their physicians and other caregivers if they anticipate problems in following prescribed treatment.

Patients should also be aware of the hospital's obligation to be reasonably efficient and equitable in providing care to other patients and the community. The hospital's rules and regulations are designed to help the hospital meet this obligation. Patients and their families are responsible for making reasonable accommodations to the needs of the hospital, other patients, medical staff, and hospital employees. Patients are responsible for providing necessary information for insurance claims and for working with the hospital to make payment arrangements, when necessary.

A person's health depends on much more than health care services. Patients are responsible for recognizing the impact of their life-style on their personal health.

## Conclusion

Hospitals have many functions to perform, including the enhancement of health status, health promotion, and the prevention and treatment of injury and disease; the immediate and ongoing care and rehabilitation of patients; the education of health professionals, patients, and the community; and research. All these activities must be conducted with an overriding concern for the values and dignity of patients.

*A Patient's Bill of Rights* was first adopted by the American Hospital Association in 1973. This revision was approved by the AHA Board of Trustees on October 21, 1992. © 1992 by the American Hospital Association, 840 North Lake Shore Drive, Chicago, Illinois 60611. Printed in the U.S.A. All rights reserved. Catalog no. 157759.

# A P P E N D I X

# B

 Examples of Legal Documents

The items found in this appendix are examples of the types of legal documents that an individual involved in a legal action may encounter.

B–1. (a,b) Release of Records Authorization: medical records may not be released without the expressed permission of the patient or legal representative unless otherwise required by law.

B–2. Civil Summons: notice that a legal action has been filed against a defendant.

B–3. Complaint: a list of the plaintiff's claims against the defendant. The complaint contains: (1) a short and plain statement of the grounds upon which the court's jurisdiction depends, (2) a statement of the claim showing that the pleader is entitled to relief, (3) a demand for judgement.

B–4. Answer: the defendant's response to the plaintiff's allegations.

B–5. Notice to take Deposition: individual witnesses to be deposed are sent a notice of deposition which identifies the individual, the time, the date, and the location of the deposition.

B–6. Subpoena Duces Tecum: A notice to a witness to bring documents (records) to a deposition or other hearing.

B–7. Notice of authentication of records: In order to authenticate original or copies of medical records, the custodian of the records is generally called to testify. In many jurisdictions, the custodian is able to enter a signed affidavit which authenticates the records in lieu of appearing in court.

**B–1(a)**

---

### RELEASE OF RECORDS AUTHORIZATION

Month, day, year

Hospital X
Elm Street
Anywhere, USA

I, Patient A, hereby authorize the physician(s), hospital, or clinic to furnish full and complete medical reports, billing statements, and information requested by the undersigned, to Ann M. Obergfell, attorney-at-law or any representative from her office; this authorization includes examination of all hospital records, x-ray film, and furnishing of any information including opinions or interpretations.

Your full cooperation with my attorney or her representatives is requested. You are further requested to disclose no information to any other person without further written authority. All prior authorization is hereby cancelled.

_____
patient's name

_____
address

State of _____

County of _____

Subscribed and sworn to before me by _____,

this _____ day of _____, 199____.

My commission expires: _____

_____
Notary Public, State at Large

**B–1(b)**

## AUTHORIZATION FOR MEDICAL REPORTS, HOSPITAL RECORDS, WAGE RECORDS, AND MISCELLANEOUS RECORDS

Name _____  Address _____

Date of Birth _____  SS# _____

Type Case _____  Date of Incident _____

To Whom It May Concern:

I hereby authorize Ann M. Obergfell, or the bearer hereof, to inspect and copy any and all medical reports, hospital records, prescription files, drug records, wage records, and all other records of any nature, including but not restricted to those of the Social Security Administration, Internal Revenue Service, Kentucky Department of Revenue, Railroad Retirement Board, Veterans Administration and any police department records.

I further authorize and request each physician to give the bearer hereof a full medical report, including the amount of his bill.

You are further requested to disclose no information to any insurance adjuster or other persons without written authority from me to do so. All prior authorization are hereby canceled.

A photostatic copy hereof shall be considered as fully as the original.

_____

_____

_____

**B–2**

---

**Case No.** _____

### Civil Summons

Court  _____

County  _____

Patient A                    Plaintiff
1000 Main Street
Anywhere, USA                vs.

Hospital X                   Defendant
Elm Street
Anywhere, USA

To the above-named defendants:

You are hereby notified that a legal action has been filed against you in this court demanding relief as shown on the document delivered to you with this summons. Unless a written defense is made by you or by an attorney in your behalf within 20 days following the day this paper is delivered to you, judgement by default may be taken against you for the relief demanded in the attached complaint.

The name(s) and address(es) of the party or parties demanding such relief against you or the parties attorney(s) are shown on the document delivered to you with this summons.

Date: _____    Clerk: _____

### PROOF OF SERVICE

This summons was served by delivering a true copy and the complaint (or other initiating document) to: _____

_____

This _____ day of _____, 19_____.

Served by: _____

B-3

Case No. _____          Circuit Court _____

                              Division _____


## COMPLAINT


Patient A                    Plaintiff
1000 Main Street
Anywhere, USA                vs.


Hospital X                   Defendant
Elm Street
Anywhere, USA


Comes the plaintiff, patient A, by counsel, and for her complaint against the defendant herein, would show as follows:

1. That the plaintiff (patient A) is an adult resident of Anywhere, USA.
2. That the defendant, Hospital X, is a corporation located and operating in Anywhere, USA
3. That on or about May 8, 1994, the plaintiff was a patient in Hospital X.
4. That at the time above mentioned, plaintiff was caused to fall by reason of a defective condition in a section of the floor located in and immediately in front of the radiographic table located in the radiology department room 4. Said defective condition being a spilled fluid-like substance.
5. That the aforementioned floor is and has long been an area for patient travel under the sole control of the defendant.
6. It was the duty of the defendant hospital to maintain the area of patient travel in a safe condition.
7. The defendant, not regarding its duty, neglected and failed to keep said aforementioned floor in good condition and negligently allowed it to become defective and/or in an unsafe condition, all of which was known to defendant, its agents or officers, or by the

exercise of reasonable diligence or ordinary care, could have been known by them.

8. That as a result of the defendant's negligence in maintaining the floor, the plaintiff was caused to fall and to suffer bodily injuries, physical and mental pain.

9. That as a direct result of plaintiff's fall and resulting injuries, plaintiff was caused to incur expenses for and incident to medical treatment and to lose time from the transaction of her daily affairs and to suffer permanent impairment of her ability to labor and earn wages.

10. In accordance with civil procedures rules, the plaintiff's damages are in excess of any minimum dollar amount necessary to establish jurisdiction of this court and the plaintiff, patient A, seeks an amount that is fair and reasonable as shown by the evidence to compensate her for her pain and suffering, both physical and mental, the permanent impairment of her earning capacity and all further damages sustained by her.

11. That the plaintiff complied with all statutory requirements of written notice to the defendant, Hospital X, by causing such notice to be prepared and delivered within the statutorily required period to Hospital X.


WHEREFORE, plaintiff, patient a, demands judgement against the defendant, Hospital X, as follows:

1. Compensatory damages as determined to be reasonable under the evidence of her medical expense, lost wages, permanent impairment of her ability to labor and for her pain and suffering, past, present and future.

2. Trial by jury in all issues so triable.

3. Her costs herein expended.

4. All other relief to which she may be entitled.


Attorney
First Street
Anywhere, USA
COUNSEL FOR PLAINTIFF

**B–4**

Case No. _____          Circuit Court _____

                                  Division _____


### ANSWER


Patient A                    Plaintiff

                             vs.

Hospital X                   Defendant


Comes the defendant, Hospital X, by counsel and for their response to the complain filed herein, states as follows:


### FIRST DEFENSE

1. The complaint fails to state a claim upon which relief can be granted.


### SECOND DEFENSE

2. This Defendant had no prior notice of the alleged defective condition of the floor.

3. This Answering Defendant denies allegations contained in Paragraphs 7 and 8 of Plaintiff's complaint herein.

4. This Answering Defendant is without sufficient knowledge or information to form an opinion as to the truth of allegations contained in paragraphs 1, 3, 4, 5, 6, 9, 10, and 11 of plaintiff's complaint herein.

5. This Answering Defendant admits allegations contained in paragraph 2 of Plaintiff's complaint herein.

6. This Answering Defendant denies each and every allegation not specifically pled in the Complaint.

7. This Answering Defendant reserves the right to plead further as facts become known to the Defendant.


WHEREFORE, the Defendant respectfully requests that:

1. The complaint be dismissed
2. For their costs herein expended.
3. For a trial by jury
4. For any and all other relief to which they may properly be entitled.

Respectfully submitted,


Attorney for Defendant


## CERTIFICATE OF SERVICE

I hereby certify that a copy of the foregoing was mailed this _____ day of _____, 1995.

**B–5**

---

**Case No.** _____          Court _____

Division _____

### NOTICE TO TAKE DEPOSITION

TO: Attorney at Law          Attorney at Law
    Anywhere, USA          Anywhere, USA

PLEASE TAKE NOTICE that the undersigned will on Friday, February 3, 1995 at the hour of 2:00 pm, take the deposition of James Kildaire, M.D., at Hospital X, Elm Street, Anywhere, USA pursuant to and for all purposes provided for in the Rules of Civil Procedure.

_____

Attorney
Anywhere, USA

### CERTIFICATION

I hereby certify that a copy hereof was mailed to the above named person at the address listed on this the _____ day of _____, 1995.

_____

**B–6**

The State of X                    Plaintiff

vs.

John Doe                          Defendant


TO:  Medical Records Librarian
     Hospital Y
     1234 State St.
     Anywhere, USA


### Subpoena Duces Tecum


You are hereby required to furnish to the Grand Jury, any or all records, including Doctors' and or Nurses' notations, pertaining to the examination, testing, treatment, and admission of Patient _____.

ON (date): February 19, 1995
AT (time): 11:00 a.m.
          Grand Jury
          3rd Floor, Hall of Justice


to testify on behalf of the State of X as a witness in the case of the State of X, Plaintiff against the above-named defendant.
     before the Honorable Judge A.



_____
Witness:            , Circuit Court Clerk

**B–7**

Date: _____

<u>To Whom It May Concern:</u>

As custodian of the Medical Records at Hospital X, I hereby state that the enclosed medical records of Patient A, hospital number 12345, consisting of 45 pages, are true and complete reproductions of the original or microfilmed medical records which are housed at Hospital X. The original records were made in the regular course of business, and it was the regular course of Hospital X to make such records at or near the time of the matter recorded. This certification is given pursuant to KRS 422.305 in lieu of my personal appearance.

Sincerely,

Director of Medical Records
Hospital X

Acknowledged before me this _____ day of _____, 1995.

_____
Notary Public

My Commission expires _____.

# A P P E N D I X
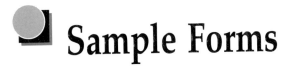

# C

# ◼ Sample Forms

Appendix C offers the reader sample forms which may be adopted or adapted to meet the needs of the individual department, clinic, or office.

## SAMPLE FORMS

A. Radiology Flow Sheet: This form is designed for use in imaging and therapy departments where invasive procedures are performed. The patient education aspect of the procedure is incorporated into the form. The patient will sign the form indicating that the procedure and the pre- and post-exam instructions were thoroughly explained. The form is then incorporated in the patient's permanent medical record.

Reprinted with permission of Baptist Hospital East, Louisville, KY.

B. Adverse Drug Reaction Reporting: Any reaction to medication should be documented in the patient record. The adverse drug reaction form can be utilized by imaging and therapy departments to assist in patient recordkeeping procedures. When a reaction is reported, documentation will be included in the nursing or radiology notes (see form C) and the drug identification card will be completed and forwarded to the pharmacy where the patient's drug sensitivity list can be updated.

Reprinted with permission of Baptist Hospital East, Louisville, KY.

C. Radiology Notes: All patient medical records include nursing notes. Some facilities do not allow radiology personnel to document in nursing notes based on a misconception that radiology personnel do not perform patient care. Since patient care is an integral part of imaging and therapy services and should be documented in the same fashion as patient care in any other area of the facility, a radiology notes page should be included in the patient's medical record.

D. Radiology History Form: Procedures in imaging and therapy departments should not be performed unless appropriate patient history and assessment is completed. Forms which allow the technologist to document pertinent history in an orderly fashion will assure that the correct information is available when determining how to complete a procedure and when the radiologist or other physician is interpreting the completed images.

Reprinted with permission Floyd Memorial Hospital, New Albany, IN.

E. Patient Information Sheet: Another example of a patient information form which is completed by the technologist and, because of the multiple copy format, is incorporated in the patient medical record, the quality review record, and the department records.

Reprinted with permission of Taylor County Hospital, Campbellsville, KY.

F. Supply Data Sheet: Departments may keep an accurate record of supplies utilized on each patient if they incorporate a miscellaneous charges form into the documentation process.

Reprinted with permission of Taylor County Hospital, Campbellsville, KY.

G. Radiographic Variance Form: The form can be used for patients entering the imaging department from the emergency room. The form can be used with each patient for history and assessment as well as follow up on variations between ER and radiology interpretation. The use of anatomic images will allow the technologist to mark areas of injury and will allow patients to point to affected areas if they are unable to speak or answer questions.

Reprinted with permission Audubon Regional Medical Center, Louisville, KY.

H. Mammography—History and Notice Form: This form can be utilized in any office, clinic, or department which provides mammographic procedures. History can be gathered from the patient and the information can be used during the interpretation stage by the radiologist. Prompt result reporting can be accomplished if the facility elects to utilize the reporting form which also offers some additional information concerning mammography for the patient.

Reprinted with permission of Floyd Memorial Hospital, New Albany, IN.

## Sample Form A

```
                    BAPTIST HOSPITAL EAST
                    RADIOLOGY FLOW SHEET
                                              ROOM #:_____

NAME:_____  HOSPITAL #: _____
DATE: _____ AGE: _____  PHYSICIAN: _____
PROCEDURE:_____  RADIOLOGIST: _____
PATIENT DENIES PREGNANCY:    YES_____  NO_____  N/A _____
PREMEDICATION: _____
ALLERGIES: _____


        IV LINE/ANGIO CATHETER              LAB RESULTS
INFUSING _____ INSERTED_____ BY_____   BUN _____  [8-20]
IV SITE  _____     CR  _____  [0.5-1.2]
NUMBER OF VENIPUNCTURE ATTEMPTS _____ (  )  PT  _____  [11.6-14]  (CONTROL 11.8)
TYPE OF NEEDLE _____   PTT _____  [25.5-34.5](CONTROL 30.0)
TIME INSERTED  _____   K+  _____  [3.5-5.0]
TIME REMOVED  _____   HGB _____  [12-14]
CONDITION : NO INFLAMMATION _____   HCT _____  [37-47]
INFLAMED _____ HEMATOMA _____    PLTS_____  [140-500]
INFILTRATED _____


URINARY CATHETER USED:  INDWELLING _____ INSERTED _____ SIZE _____
INSERTED FOR VCU    YES ___ NO___ (SEE NOTES)


CONTRAST/RADIONUCLIDE                    REACTION TO CONTRAST
TYPE 1)  _____ 2) _____    NO____ YES ____ (DESCRIBE)
LOT NO 1) _____ 2) _____    (IF SEVERE, FILL OUT
EXP DATE 1) _____ 2) _____    ADVERSE REACTION FORM)
AMOUNT 1)  _____ 2) _____


*FOR INTRAVENOUS PYELOGRAM
PATIENT DENIES RISK FACTORS   YES_____ NO_____  IF NO, STATE RISK FACTOR _____

THE ABOVE PROCEDURE HAS BEEN EXPLAINED TO ME INCLUDING PRE AND POST EXAM

INSTRUCTION. _____ PATIENT

NOTES: _____
_____
_____
_____
_____

033606 (11/94)
```

## Sample Form B

| POSSIBLE ADVERSE DRUG REACTION IDENTIFICATION CARD | |
| --- | --- |
| DRUG: | ADDRESSOGRAPH |
| DATE/REACTION: | |
| RN/LPN/DATE: | |
| REACTION:<br>☐ RASH            ☐ HEADACHE<br>☐ CHG. HEART RATE       ☐ ANAPHYLAXIS<br>☐ CHG. RENAL FUNCTION   ☐ GI DISTRESS<br>☐ ALTERED MENTAL STATE<br>☐ OTHER:<br><br><br>PHYSICIAN PLEASE CHECK APPROPRIATE BOX:<br>   ☐ ADVERSE DRUG REACTION<br>   ☐ *NOT* AN ADVERSE DRUG REACTION<br>PHYSICIAN<br>SIGNATURE _____ | |
| **NOT PART OF PERMANENT RECORD** | |
| **RETURN TO THE PHARMACY** | |

Sample Form C

| DATE | RADIOLOGY NOTES |
|------|------------------|
|      |                  |
|      |                  |
|      |                  |
|      |                  |
|      |                  |
|      |                  |
|      |                  |
|      |                  |
|      |                  |
|      |                  |
|      |                  |
|      |                  |
|      |                  |
|      |                  |
|      |                  |
|      |                  |
|      |                  |
|      |                  |
|      |                  |
|      |                  |
|      |                  |
|      |                  |

## Sample Form D

---

### RADIOLOGY HISTORY FORM

**P A T I E N T**

**I N F O**

NAME _____ AGE _____ DATE _____

RADIOLOGY NUMBER _____ TECHNOLOGIST NUMBER _____

REFERRING DOCTOR _____

HISTORY FROM DOCTORS: _____

_____

EXAM EXPLAINED:   YES    NO    (*circle one*)

QUESTIONS/CONCERNS: _____

_____

1. Date of last menstrual period: _____

2. Are you on birth control pills?   YES    NO    (*circle one*)

3. Have you had a tubal ligation or hysterectomy?    YES    NO
                                                   (*circle one*)

4. Is there a possibility that you may be pregnant?  YES    NO
                                                   (*circle one*)
   _____ (*Signature*)

---

**C H E S T**

**H I S T O R Y**

Patient's History: (*check all that apply*)
Chest x-ray:  Do you currently smoke?       ☐ No  ☐ Yes
              Have you ever smoked?          ☐ No  ☐ Yes
              Has it been 5 years since quitting?  ☐ No  ☐ Yes

| | |
|---|---|
| ☐ COUGH | ☐ HEART DISEASE |
| ☐ FEVER | ☐ HIGH BLOOD PRESSURE |
| ☐ CONGESTION | ☐ PNEUMONIA |
| ☐ COUGHING BLOOD | ☐ TUBERCULOSIS |
| ☐ SHORT OF BREATH | ☐ PNEUMOTHORAX |
| ☐ CHEST PAIN | ☐ BROKEN RIBS |
| ☐ MI (MYOCARDIAL INFARCTION) | ☐ CANCER |
| ☐ HEART FAILURE | ☐ OTHER _____ |

---

**E X T R E M I T Y**

**H I S T O R Y**

EXTREMITY:   RT ☐   LT ☐   BODY PART _____

HISTORY: _____

_____

_____

_____

130048 (11/93)

GI HISTORY

FLUOROSCOPY:    ☐ UGI    ☐ SMALL BOWEL    ☐ COLON

☐ NAUSEA
☐ VOMITING
☐ BLOOD    ☐ EMESIS    ☐ STOOL
☐ PAIN
☐ BLOATING OR DISTENSION
☐ DIARRHEA
☐ CONSTIPATION

☐ ULCER    WHEN _____
☐ CANCER    SITE _____
        WHEN _____

☐ SURGERY - OTHER THAN CANCER
        WHY _____
        WHEN _____
☐ ULCERATIVE COLITIS
☐ CROHN'S DISEASE

IVP HISTORY

IVP: ALLERGIES  ☐ YES  ☐ NO    SPECIFY _____
PREVIOUS CONTRAST REACTIONS: _____

☐ KIDNEY FAILURE        BUN _____    CR _____
☐ CANCER _____ KIDNEY _____ BLADDER _____ OTHER
☐ HISTORY OF KIDNEY STONES
☐ PAIN    RT    LT
☐ FEVER
☐ DIFFICULTY IN URINATION

☐ BLOOD
☐ BLADDER INFECTION
☐ OTHER

SITE:   RIGHT ANTECUBITAL, LEFT ANTECUBITAL, IV TUBING
    OTHER _____
DIFFICULTY IN ADMINISTRATION?    YES    NO
EXPLAIN IF YES: _____
BLOOD RETURN SEEN?    YES    NO

MYELOGRAM:    CERVICAL ☐        THORACIC ☐        LUMBAR ☐

        PUNCTURE SITE _____

CONSENT OBTAINED:  YES ☐    NO ☐
IF NO, EXPLAIN REASON: _____
_____
_____

VENOGRAM:    RT ☐    LT ☐    ARM ☐    LEG ☐

CONTRAST USED:    TYPE: _____

        AMOUNT: _____

CONSENT OBTAINED:  YES ☐    NO ☐
IF NO, EXPLAIN REASON: _____
_____
_____

        PUNCTURE SITE _____

# Sample Form E

**TAYLOR COUNTY HOSPITAL**     MEDICAL RECORDS

NAME:

MEDICAL RECORDS NO.:                     **RADIOLOGY**

AGE:    SEX:    DOB:

DATE OF STUDY:             PROCEDURE:

LOCATION:              ACCOUNT NO.:

**SPECIAL INSTRUCTIONS:**      ORDER NO.:

1                      DATE OF ORDER:

2                      TIME OF ORDER:

3                      ENT. FROM:

4 ALLERGIES            ENT. BY:

5 MODE OF TRAN.        REQUESTING

**PERTINENT CLINICAL DATA:**     DOCTOR:

**FILM COUNT**

| 14 x 17 | **DIGITAL** | **DUPLICATING** |
|---|---|---|
| 10 x 12 | 11 x 14 | 14 x 17 |
| 8 x 10 | 8 x 10 | 10 x 12 |
| 11 x 14 | **MAMMO** | **TAPE** |
| 9 x 9 | 10 x 12 | **OTHER** |
| 7 x 17 | 8 x 10 | |

| **RADIOLOGY CHECKLIST** | Y | N | N/A |
|---|---|---|---|
| PATIENT IDENTIFIED | | | |
| PROCEDURE IDENTIFIED | | | |
| PREGNANCY STATUS | | | |
| INFORMED CONSENT COMPLETED | | | |
| EXAMINATION COMPLETED | | | |
| EXAMINATION RESCHEDULED | | | |
| D/C INSTRUCTIONS GIVEN | | | |
| CONDITION UNCHANGED AT D/C | | | |
| UNEXPECTED OUTCOMES | | | |

**STATISTICS**

TIME IN:

EXAMINATION TIME:

TIME OUT:

EXAMINATION ROOM:

FLUOROSCOPY TIME:

RECEPTIONIST:

RADIOLOGIST:

TECHNOLOGIST:

OTHER:

**TREATMENT (PROCEDURES)**

CLEANSING ENEMA AT        BY

**URINARY CATHETER:**    SIZE    TIME    BY

    ☐ FOLEY

    ☐ STRAIGHT

**SKIN PREPARATION:** AREA: _____

SHAVE PREP           BY

BETADINE SCRUB.       BY

**OTHER:**

**DISPOSITION**

| **LOCATION** | FROM | TO |
|---|---|---|
| INPATIENT ROOM | | |
| OUTPATIENT | | |
| OUTPATIENT SURGERY | | |
| ER | | |
| ICU | | |
| SURGERY | | |
| OB | | |
| DOCTOR'S OFFICE | | |
| HOME | | |
| OTHER | | |
| **MOBILITY STATUS** | | |
| SELF | | |
| ASSISTANCE | | |
| IMMOBILE | | |
| OTHER | | |
| **MODE OF TRANSPORT** | | |
| AMBULATORY | | |
| WHEELCHAIR | | |
| STRETCHER | | |
| CARRIED | | |
| PORTABLE | | |
| OTHER | | |
| **PATIENT STATUS** | | |
| ALERT | | |
| ORIENTED | | |
| CONFUSED | | |
| AGITATED | | |
| LETHARGIC/DROWSY | | |
| NON-RESPONSIVE | | |
| OTHER | | |

**VITAL SIGNS**

| TIME | PULSE | BLOOD PRESSURE |
|---|---|---|
| | | |
| | | |
| | | |
| | | |
| | | |
| | | |
| | | |
| | | |
| | | |
| | | |
| | | |
| | | |

**MEDICINE ADMINISTRATION RECORD:**

ALLERGY HISTORY:

SOURCE: PT.      RECORDS      OTH.

MEDICATION:

ROUTE:

AMOUNT:

TIME:

BY:

BODY WT.:

OTHER:

**IV**

SIZE:            TYPE:

LOCATION:         BY:

SOLUTION:    TIME     EXISTING

NS FLUSH

**LAB RESULTS**

BUN:          CREATININE:

OTHER:

APPROVED BY:             M.D.

$O_2$       L/MIN.    CARDIAC MONITOR

**Respiratory Rate:**      **Other:**

Pulse Oximeter        Rt. ↑ Ext. ☐    Rt. ↓ Ext. ☐

Average:            Lt. ↑ Ext. ☐    Lt. ↓ Ext. ☐

Blood Pressure Cuff:    Rt. ↑ Ext. ☐    Rt. ↓ Ext. ☐

Manual ☐   Auto ☐    Lt. ↑ Ext. ☐    Lt. ↓ Ext. ☐

INSTRUCTIONS AND/OR COMMENTS: _____

EMERGENCY DEPT. INTERPRETATION: _____

AGREE: ☐      CORRECTION: ☐

EMERGENCY ROOM PHYSICIAN: _____

STAFF PHYSICIAN: _____

RADIOLOGISTS: _____

NOTIFIED:_____ DATE: _____ TIME: _____

BY: _____

# Sample Form F

**TAYLOR COUNTY HOSPITAL**
NAME:
MEDICAL RECORDS NO.:
AGE:    SEX:    DOB:
DATE OF STUDY:
LOCATION:
    SPECIAL INSTRUCTIONS:
1
2
3
4 ALLERGIES
5 MODE OF TRAN.
PERTINENT CLINICAL DATA:

SUPPLY DATA

PROCEDURE:
ACCOUNT NO.:
ORDER NO.:
DATE OF ORDER:
TIME OF ORDER:
ENT. FROM:
ENT. BY:
REQUESTING
DOCTOR:

## RADIOLOGY

## RADIOLOGY MISCELLANEOUS CHARGES

| SOLUTIONS | 250 | 500 | 1000 | 1500 | |
|---|---|---|---|---|---|
| D5LR | | 475-20036 | 475-20037 | | |
| Dextrose | 475-20012 | 475-20013 | 475-20016 | | |
| H20 Irrigation | | | | 475-20092 | |
| Lactated Ringers | 475-20050 | 475-20055 | 475-20058 | | |
| Normal Saline | 475-20082 | 475-20021 | 475-20085 | | |
| D5 ½ NS | | 475-20032 | 475-20034 | | |
| ½ NS | | 475-20095 | 475-20099 | | |
| NS Irrigation | | 475-20088 | | 475-20091 | |
| Other | | | | | |

| MEDICATIONS | | IV EQUIPMENT | |
|---|---|---|---|
| Benadryl 25 m. | | Angio Catheter 22 ga. | 421-30004 |
| Benadryl 50 mg. | 475-132 | Angio Catheter 14-20 ga. | 421-30001 |
| Bowel Prep Kit | 475-349 | Angio-Set 22-18 ga. | 421-30002 |
| Chloral Hydrate 500 mg. | 475-200 | IV Care Kit | 421-50463 |
| Fleets Enema Kit | 421-50331 | J-Loop Connector | 421-30017 |
| Glucagon 1 Kit | 475-377 | VenoSet - Anesthesia | 421-30037 |
| Heparin Flush | 475-979 | VenoTube 30″ | 421-30057 |
| Heparin 5000 Units | 475-388 | | |
| Kinevac | 475-472 | DRESSINGS/BANDAGES | |
| Lasix 20 mg. | 475-491 | Abdomen Pad | 421-50004 |
| Lasix 40 mg. | 475-492 | Kerlex | 421-50469 |
| Lidocaine Viscous 30mls | 475-1526 | Kling 2″ | 421-50496 |
| Lidocaine 1% 10mls | 475-1895 | Kling 4″ | 421-50502 |
| Omnipaque 240 20cc | 475-1886 | 4 x 4 Packages | 421-50874 |
| Omnipaque 240 100cc | 475-1885 | 4 x 4 Tray | 421-50883 |
| Omnipaque 300 50cc | 475-1640 | | |
| Omnipaque 300 150cc | 475-1848 | | |
| Phenergan 25 mg. | 475-653 | | |
| Phenergan 50 mg. | 475-654 | | |

| MISCELLANEOUS | | | |
|---|---|---|---|
| Bedpan | 421-50075 | Minor Prep Shave | 421-50730 |
| Bile Bag | 421-50087 | PRN Adapter | 421-50720 |
| Catheter Tray | 421-10034 | Salem Sump | 421-50775 |
| Catheter Urinary | 421-10037 | Scapel | 421-50781 |
| Chux Pads | 421-50187 | Sterile Gloves | 421-50397 |
| Dobbhoff | 421-50258 | Sterile Specimen Cup | 421-50832 |
| EKG Electrode | 421-50312 | Stop Cock | 421-50934 |
| Emesis Basin | 421-50320 | Suction Catheter | 421-10046 |
| Enema Kit | 421-50331 | Suture Removal Set | 421-50967 |
| General Prep Kit | 421-50721 | Urinal | 421-51083 |
| Irrigation Tray | 421-50451 | Yaunker Tip | 421-51147 |

## Sample Form G

**Audubon Regional Medical Center**
**RADIOGRAPHIC VARIANCE**

NAME:

Technologist: _____

MED. REC. NUMBER-

Patient History:

EXAM:

(or use Phamis label)

ER PHYSICIAN INTERPRETATION:
NEGATIVE _____
OTHER:

INITIALS _____

RADIOLOGIST'S INTERPRETATION:
AGREE _____
ESSENTIALLY AGREE W/        COMMENTS:
ADDITIONAL COMMENTS _____
DISAGREE _____

INITIALS _____

**IF THE RADIOLOGIST DISAGREES WITH EMERGENCY ROOM PHYSICIAN, PROMPTLY NOTIFY THE EMERGENCY DEPARTMENT.**

PERSON NOTIFIED (NAME) _____
BY (NAME) _____     TIME _____
DATE _____

**EMERGENCY DEPARTMENT FOLLOW UP OF X-RAY VARIANCE**
CLINICALLY SIGNIFICANT VARIANCE?:   ___ yes   ___ no   ___ If no, Why: _____
CHANGE IN MEDICAL CARE REQUIRED:   ___ yes   ___ no   ___ If yes, specify additional evaluation/treatments.
_____

NOTIFICATION:   ___ M.D. (Name) _____
                       Date _____
               ___ PT. (Name) _____
                       Date _____
               ___ Certified Letter Sent (Attach copy) Date _____
FOLLOW UP:   ___ Pt. to follow up to PMD for additional treatment/evaluation
             ___ Pt. to follow-up with ED for additional treatment/evaluation

SIGNATURE: _____ DATE/TIME _____

WHITE - MEDICAL RECORDS          PINK - ED          YELLOW - RADIOLOGY

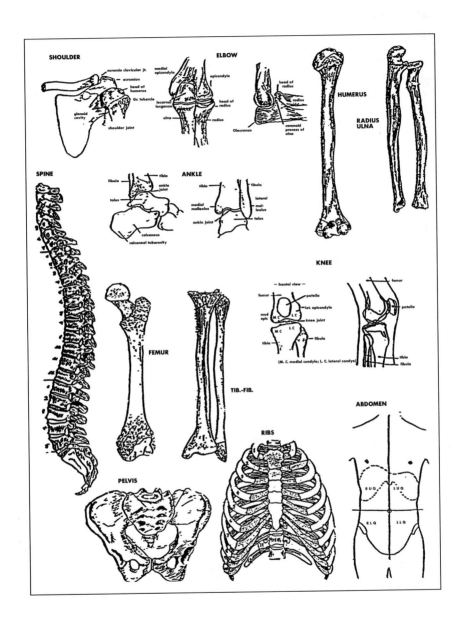

# Sample Form H

**Floyd Memorial Hospital**
1850 State Street, New Albany, Indiana 47150 (812)948-7791

Date:_____

ACR
ACCREDITED

**Diagnostic Breast Center**
A Service of Floyd Memorial Hospital

Thank you for using the Diagnostic Breast Center of Floyd Memorial Hospital. A copy of your mammogram report has been forwarded to your physician,

Dr. _____.

The report of your mammogram exam was:

☐ Normal. The next recommended mammogram should be in _____ years.

☐ The report of your mammogram indicates you should consult your physician. The report indicates a need for further follow-up.

Patient Name _____

Address _____

City, State, Zip _____

If we can be of further assistance, please call (812)948-7409.
For your information: Your mammogram films are included in your radiographic file at this location.
There is at least a 15% false negative rate in mammographic detection of cancer. Therefore, management of a palpable abnormality must be based on clinical grounds and a negative mammography report should not defer further breast evaluation when clinically indicated.
Importance of mammography: We feel that screening mammography is beneficial in early detection of breast cancer. Screening mammography should therefore be part of an annual health maintenance program. This should include annual physical exam by your physician and monthly self breast examinations.
It is the patient's responsibility to inform any new doctor or mammography center of the date and place of her previous mammogram.

· Procedure Explained?  ☐ Yes  ☐ No     Comment:_____

· Are you pregnant?  ☐ Yes  ☐ No     If yes, inform technologist.     Last menstrual period _____

_____ (Signature)  Age: _____

· Previous mammogram?  ☐ Yes  ☐ No   Where?_____ When? _____

Results of previous mammogram?_____

· Have you ever had breast surgery?   ☐ Yes  ☐ No

What type?  Biopsy:       Right ☐   Year _____      Left ☐   Year _____
           Lumpectomy:   Right ☐   Year _____      Left ☐   Year _____
           Mastectomy:   Right ☐   Year _____      Left ☐   Year _____
           Other _____
           Any radiation treatment: _____
           Results of above: _____

· What is the reason for today's exam?     ☐ Screening          ☐ Other

· Any problems with your breasts?   ☐ Yes  ☐ No    If yes, is it:  Lump ☐      Right ☐   Left ☐
                                                              Discharge ☐  Right ☐   Left ☐   Color of Discharge _____
                                                              Pain ☐       Right ☐   Left ☐ _____
                                                              Other ☐      Right ☐   Left ☐   Explain: _____

· Have either your mother or sister had breast cancer before age 50?   ☐ Yes  ☐ No   If yes, Mother ☐   Sister ☐

· Are you taking female hormones or birth control pills?   ☐ Yes  ☐ No   When did you start? _____

FOR STAFF USE ONLY

| | KV | MAS | DENS | CM |
|---|---|---|---|---|
| Rt CC | KV _____ | MAS _____ | DENS _____ | CM _____ |
| Rt MLO | KV _____ | MAS _____ | DENS _____ | CM _____ |
| Lt CC | KV _____ | MAS _____ | DENS _____ | CM _____ |
| Lt MLO | KV _____ | MAS _____ | DENS _____ | CM _____ |
| | KV _____ | MAS _____ | DENS _____ | CM _____ |
| | KV _____ | MAS _____ | DENS _____ | CM _____ |

Right Lateral     Right Frontal     Left Frontal     Left Lateral

_____ BC1     _____ BC2

X-ray No. _____     Tech: _____

**Floyd Memorial Hospital**
1850 State Street, New Albany, Indiana 47150 (812)944-7701

Date:_____

ACR
ACCREDITED

**Diagnostic Breast Center**
A Service of Floyd Memorial Hospital

Thank you for using the Diagnostic Breast Center of Floyd Memorial Hospital.  A copy of your mammogram report has been forwarded to your physician,

Dr. _____.

The report of your mammogram exam was:

☐ Normal.  The next recommended mammogram should be in _____ years.

☐ The report of your mammogram indicates you should consult your physician.  The report indicates a need for further follow-up.

Patient Name _____

Address _____

City, State, Zip _____

If we can be of further assistance, please call (812)948-7409.
For your information:  Your mammogram films are included in your radiographic file at this location.
There is at least a 15% false negative rate in mammographic detection of cancer.  Therefore, management of a palpable abnormality must be based on clinical grounds and a negative mammography report should not defer further breast evaluation when clinically indicated.
Importance of mammography:  We feel that screening mammography is beneficial in early detection of breast cancer.  Screening mammography should therefore be part of an annual health maintenance program.  This should include annual physical exam by your physician and monthly self breast examinations.
It is the patient's responsibility to inform any new doctor or mammography center of the date and place of her previous mammogram.

# A P P E N D I X
# D

## ADDITIONAL OSHA (GENERAL INDUSTRY) STANDARDS FOR REVIEW

29 CFR 1910.1000    Air contaminants
29 CFR 1910.1030    Bloodborne Pathogens
29 CFR 1910.333    Electrical Safety–related Work Practices
29 CFR 1910.151    Emergency Flushing, Eyes and Body
29 CFR 1910.157    Fire Protection
29 CFR 1910.1200    Hazard Communication
29 CFR 1910.120    Hazardous Waste Operations (Emergency Response)
29 CFR 1910.151    Medical Services and First Aid
29 CFR 1910.96,.97    Radiation—Employee Exposure

Recommended reading:

1. National Institute for Occupational Safety and Health. *Guidelines for Protecting the Safety and Health of Health Care Workers.* PB89-1148621 (September 1988).
2. American Conference of Governmental Industrial Hygienists (ACGIH). *1993–1994 Threshold Limit Values for Chemical Substances and Physical Agents and Biological Exposure Indices.*
3. *Memorandum of Understanding Between the Occupational Safety and Health Administration and the Nuclear Regulatory Commission.* 53 Federal Register 43950, amended by OSHA Instruction CPL 2.86 (22 December 1989).

29 CFR 1910.96    Ionizing Radiation Standard
Generally the NRC licenses and regulates the use of radioactive materials, while OSHA regulations cover hazards produced by x-ray machines and other types of atomic accelerators.

29 CFR 1910.97     Nonionizing Radiation

Ultrasound, visible radiation (lasers), ultraviolet radiation, radiofrequency/microwave, and infrared radiation are not regulated under a specific OSHA standard. However, recommendations have been issued by other organizations, such as NIOSH and the American Conference of Governmental Industrial Hygienists.

## SAMPLE SAFETY CHECKLIST

The following list is intended as a guide to be used to develop a facility-specific safety checklist.

| YES | NO | SAMPLE SAFETY CHECKLIST |
|-----|-----|-------------------------|
| | | **1. Walking and Working Surfaces** |
| ___ | ___ | Are surfaces clean, dry, and free from obstruction? (29 CFR 1910.22) |
| | | **2. Storage** |
| ___ | ___ | Are storage areas clean, dry, and stocked with lightest objects on top shelves and heavier objects on lower shelves? |
| ___ | ___ | Are outside cardboard cartons removed from the area? |
| ___ | ___ | Are fire regulations considered in storage areas? (29 CFR 1910.22) |
| | | **3. Lighting** |
| ___ | ___ | Is adequate light provided in all work areas? |
| | | **4. Exits (for evacuation)** |
| ___ | ___ | Are exits marked and free from obstruction? |
| | | **5. Fire Prevention and Protection** |
| ___ | ___ | Are fire extinguishers the appropriate type and fully charged? Are they inspected annually? |
| ___ | ___ | Are evacuation signs posted? |
| ___ | ___ | Have employees received annual training in fire safety? (NFPA 101 Life Safety Code) |
| | | **6. Hazardous Materials** |
| ___ | ___ | Are all hazardous materials identified on a department list? |
| ___ | ___ | Are hazardous materials stored properly? |
| ___ | ___ | Have employees received appropriate training on how to read and interpret information on product labels and Material Safety Data Sheets (MSDS)? |
| ___ | ___ | Have employees received appropriate training for use of hazardous materials? |
| ___ | ___ | Are employees prohibited from eating in areas where toxic materials are present? |
| ___ | ___ | Are suitable facilities available for quick flushing of the eyes and skin when a person has been exposed to corrosive material? Refer to MSDS for all products used in the department. (29 CFR 1910.1200) |

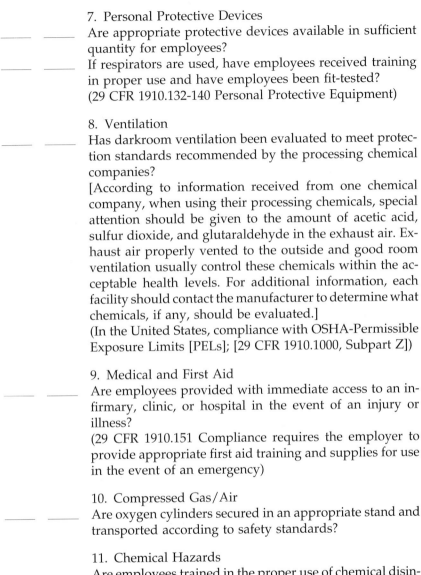

7. Personal Protective Devices

_____    _____   Are appropriate protective devices available in sufficient quantity for employees?

_____    _____   If respirators are used, have employees received training in proper use and have employees been fit-tested? (29 CFR 1910.132-140 Personal Protective Equipment)

8. Ventilation

_____    _____   Has darkroom ventilation been evaluated to meet protection standards recommended by the processing chemical companies?

[According to information received from one chemical company, when using their processing chemicals, special attention should be given to the amount of acetic acid, sulfur dioxide, and glutaraldehyde in the exhaust air. Exhaust air properly vented to the outside and good room ventilation usually control these chemicals within the acceptable health levels. For additional information, each facility should contact the manufacturer to determine what chemicals, if any, should be evaluated.]

(In the United States, compliance with OSHA-Permissible Exposure Limits [PELs]; [29 CFR 1910.1000, Subpart Z])

9. Medical and First Aid

_____    _____   Are employees provided with immediate access to an infirmary, clinic, or hospital in the event of an injury or illness?

(29 CFR 1910.151 Compliance requires the employer to provide appropriate first aid training and supplies for use in the event of an emergency)

10. Compressed Gas/Air

_____    _____   Are oxygen cylinders secured in an appropriate stand and transported according to safety standards?

11. Chemical Hazards

_____    _____   Are employees trained in the proper use of chemical disinfectants?

Commonly used disinfectants that pose a hazard to health care workers include isopropyl alcohol, ethyl alcohol, chlorine (sodium hypochlorite), iodine, and phenolics. (29 CFR 1910.1047)

[_Special note:_ While most radiographers are not in contact with ethylene oxide (used as a chemical sterilant for heat-sensitive medical instruments), employees need to understand the importance of proper work practice and engineering controls.]

_____ _____ Are employees trained in the proper use and work practices for glutaraldehyde (primarily used as a disinfectant for cold sterilization of medical instruments)?
Common products that contain glutaraldehyde include Cidex, Wavicide, Metricide, and Omnicide.
[*Special note:* Glutaraldehyde is also found in processing chemicals. Refer to the MSDS for safe work practices and protective equipment.]

_____ _____ Are employees trained in the use of equipment containing mercury and mercury spill procedures? Although much of the equipment today uses less toxic alternatives, some thermometers and sphygmomanometers still contain mercury, so proper work practice controls are needed. (29 CFR 1910.1000)

12. Infection Control and Employee Health
_____ _____ Are the following infection control practices used by all employees?
a. Universal precautions
b. Safer needle devices (when applicable)
c. Proper handwashing techniques
d. Appropriate personal protective equipment
_____ _____ Is there an exposure control plan in place to meet the standards for bloodborne pathogens?
(29 CFR 1910.1030)
[*Special note:* Refer to state or local restrictions on HIV/ AIDS policy to determine if more restrictive policies are required.]
_____ _____ Have guidelines been established for tuberculosis infection control?

13. Signs and Labels
_____ _____ Are radiation signs located in appropriate locations?
_____ _____ Are signs indicating what to do if the patient is pregnant visible to the public?
_____ _____ Are all containers marked with the appropriate labels?

# DIRECTORY

OSHA—Occupational Safety and Health Administration
200 Constitution Avenue N.W.
Washington, DC 20210
Public Information: (202) 219-8151
OSHA Regional Offices:

Region I      Connecticut, Maine, Massachusetts, New Hampshire, Rhode Island, Vermont
              Regional Administrator
              133 Portland St., 1st Floor
              Boston, MA 02114
              (617) 565-7164

Region II     Canal Zone, New Jersey, New York, Puerto Rico, Virgin Islands
              Regional Administrator
              201 Varick St., Room 670
              New York, NY 10014
              (212) 337-2378

Region III    Delaware, District of Columbia, Maryland, Pennsylvania, Virginia, West Virginia
              Regional Administrator
              3535 Market St., Suite 2100
              Philadelphia, PA 19104
              (215) 596-1201

Region IV     Alabama, Florida, Georgia, Kentucky, Mississippi, North Carolina, South Carolina, Tennessee
              Regional Administrator
              1375 Peachtree St. N.E., Suite 587
              Atlanta, GA 30367
              (404) 347-3573

Region V      Illinois, Indiana, Michigan, Minnesota, Ohio, Wisconsin
              Regional Administrator
              230 S. Dearborn St., Room 3244
              Chicago, IL 60604
              (312) 353-2220

Region VI     Arkansas, Louisiana, New Mexico, Oklahoma, Texas
              Regional Administrator
              525 Griffin St., Room 602
              Dallas, TX 75202
              (214) 767-4731

Region VII    Iowa, Kansas, Missouri, Nebraska
              Regional Administrator

911 Walnut St., Room 406
Kansas City, MO 64106
(816) 426-5861

Region VIII    Colorado, Montana, North Dakota, South Dakota, Utah,
Wyoming
Regional Administrator
1576 Federal Bldg.
1961 Stout St.
Denver, CO 80294
(303) 844-3061

Region IX    American Samoa, Arizona, California, Guam, Hawaii,
Nevada, Trust Territory of the Pacific
Regional Administrator
71 Stevenson St., Suite 420
San Francisco, CA 94105
(415) 744-6670

Region X    Alaska, Idaho, Oregon, Washington
Regional Administrator
1111 3rd Avenue, Suite 715
Seattle, WA 98101-3212
(206) 553-5930

EPA—Environmental Protection Agency
Waterside Mall, 401 M St. S.W.
Washington, DC 20460
Agency Locater Service (202) 260-2090
EPA HOTLINE—HazMat Issues 1-800-424-9346
EPA Regional Offices include the same areas as indicated in OSHA Regional Offices. Only the telephone numbers are included in this section.

Region I       (617) 565-3400
Region II      (212) 264-2525
Region III     (215) 597-9814
Revion IV      (404) 347-4727
Region V       (312) 886-3000
Region VI      (214) 655-2100
Region VII     (913) 551-7006
Region VIII    (303) 293-1616
Region IX      (415) 744-1001
Region X       (206) 553-1234

NIOSH— National Institute for Occupational Safety and Health
Hubert H. Humphrey Bldg.
200 Independence Ave. S.W., Room 714-B
Washington, DC 20201
(202) 690-7134
Technical Information and Assistance 1-800-35-NIOSH

NRC—  Nuclear Regulatory Commission
One White Flint North Building
11555 Rockville Pike
Rockville, MD 20852
Mailing Address: Washington, DC 20555
Public Information—(202) 634-3273
Publication Information—(202) 492-7333

ACGIH—American Conference of Governmental Industrial Hygienists
6500 Glenway Avenue, Bldg. D-7
Cincinnati, OH 45211
(513) 661-7881

CDC—  Centers for Disease Control and Prevention
1600 Clifton Road NE
Atlanta, Ga 30333
Office of Health and Safety (404) 639-2172
Morbidity and Mortality Weekly Report Branch (404) 639-2104
Public Health Publications Branch (404) 639-2100
Radiation Studies Branch (404) 488-7040
Division of HIV/AIDS (404) 639-2000

AMA—  American Medical Association
Department of Environmental, Public and Occupational Health
515 North State Street
Chicago, IL 60610
(202) 737-8300

JCAHO—Joint Commission on Accreditation of Healthcare Organizations
One Renaissance Boulevard
Oakbrook Terrace, IL 60181

NFPA—  National Fire Protection Association
470 Batterymarch Park
P.O. Box 9101
Quincy, MS 02169-9101
(617) 770-3000

NSC—  National Safety Council
444 North Michigan Avenue
Chicago, IL 60611
(312) 527-4800

RCRA—  Resource Conservation and Recovery Act
This act refers to Hazardous Waste Management, refer to 40 CFR 22. RCRA provides "cradle-to-grave" authority to control hazardous wastes from generation to disposal. Enforcement of RCRA requirements lies with EPA. States may also have authority to enforce RCRA requirements.

Generators of mixed waste containing both radioactive and hazardous components should review RCRA Section 3004(j) of the Federal Register published in late Winter 1993 or Spring 1994 for more updated information.

UL—    Underwriters Laboratories, Inc.
333 Pfingsten Road
Northbrook, IL 60062
(708) 272-8800

# E

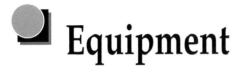

# Equipment

## OBTAINING MEDWATCH FORMS AND INSTRUCTIONS

To obtain MedWatch Form 3500 (Voluntary Reporting) and the *FDA Desk Guide to Reporting Adverse Events and Product Problems,* call 1-800-FDA-1088. The *Desk Guide* includes several copies of the form, as well as step-by-step instructions.

Bulk copies of Form 3500 may be obtained by writing to:
 Consolidated Forms and Publications Distribution Center
 Washington Commerce Center
 3222 Hubbard Road
 Landover, MD 20785

To receive up to ten copies of form 3500A, with instructions and codes for completing the form, call the Division of Small Manufacturers Assistance at 1-800-638-2041, or write to:
 Division of Small Manufacturers Assistance (HFZ-220)
 Office of Training and Assistance
 FDA/CDRH
 5600 Fishers Lane
 Rockville, MD 20857

## DEVICES TO BE TRACKED AS OF AUGUST 29, 1993

## Permanently Implantable Devices

Vascular graft prosthesis of less than 6mm diameter
Vascular graft prosthesis of 6mm and greater diameter
Total temporomandibular joint prosthesis
Glenoid fossa prosthesis
Mandibular condyle prosthesis
Interarticular disc prosthesis (interpositional implant)
Ventricular bypass (assist) device
Implantable pacemaker pulse generator
Cardiovascular permanent pacemaker electrode
Annuloplasty ring
Replacement heart valve
Automatic implantable cardioverter/defibrillor
Tracheal prosthesis
Implanted cerebellar stimulator
Implanted diaphragmatic/phrenic nerve stimulator
Implantable infusion pump

## Life-sustaining or Life-supporting Devices

Breathing frequency monitor (apnea monitor) including ventilatory efforts monitor
Continuous ventilator
DC defibrillator and paddles

## FDA-designated Devices

Silicone inflatable breast prosthesis
Silicone gel–filled breast prosthesis
Silicone gel–filled testicular prosthesis
Silicone gel–filled chin prosthesis
Silicone gel–filled Angelchik reflux valve
Infusion pump (electromechanical)

Additional information on device tracking can be found in 21 CFR 821.20.

# A P P E N D I X
# F

The information found in Appendix F can be utilized when developing an in-service and evaluation system for the facility.

F–1. Sample annual in-service plan

F–2. Sample in-service plan with objectives

F–3. Sample quiz to be used with program

F–4. (a–c) Sample competency/credentialing plan

Reprinted with permission Taylor County Hospital, Campbellsville, KY

F–5. Sample Skill Evaluation Instrument

F–1

## DEPARTMENT ANNUAL IN-SERVICE PROGRAM SCHEDULE

Each of these programs has been or will be approved for continuing education credit. Each employee is responsible for maintaining a record of continuing education credits completed. Each technologist will have an opportunity to attend the scheduled programs.

| | |
|---|---|
| January | Contrast Material Update<br>Speaker: Commercial Representative |
| February | Radiation Safety Update<br>Speaker: Department Radiation Safety Officer |
| March | Risk Management Issues in Imaging<br>Speaker: Hospital Risk Manager |
| April | Film Quality Review<br>Speaker: Quality Assurance Technologist |
| May | Safety Training Program<br>Speaker: Facility Safety Officer |
| June | Review of Departmental Protocols and Procedures<br>Speaker: Department Administrative Director |
| July | Maintaining a Positive Attitude about Patient Care<br>Speaker: Patient Education Coordinator |
| August | CPR Recertification<br>Speaker: Qualified Instructor |
| September | Equipment Update: The c-arm can be your friend<br>Speaker: Surgery Technologist<br>          Application Specialist |
| October | Trauma Radiography Review<br>Speaker: Staff Technologist |
| November | Patient's Rights and Informed Consent<br>Speaker: Facility Legal Counsel |
| December | Maintaining Department Morale<br>Speaker: Staff Technologists |

**F–2**

---

## SAFETY TRAINING PROGRAM

**15–18 Hours**                    **Hospital and Department Specific**

The safety training program is designed to acquaint employees with the protocols and procedures which when practiced will create a safer and healthier work environment.

At the completion of the training program, the employee will:

A. Identify and Practice Code Procedures
   1. Identify code names for the following conditions:
      a. fire
      b. tornado
      c. cardiac arrest
      d. ETO spill
      e. disruptive behavior
      f. internal disasters
      g. external disasters
      h. evacuation plan
   2. Describe briefly what each code means and discuss how each one impacts the facility and the employees.
   3. Discuss the role of the employee in each procedure for codes listed in the first objective.
   4. Demonstrate competence in one (randomly selected) code drill application.
   5. Explain the rationale for drill procedures for codes.
   6. Discuss the meaning of the acronyms RACE and PASS in the fire safety plan and describe the steps for how each is used.
B. Describe the Components and Use of the Hazard Communication Plan
   1. Explain the need for a Hazard Communication Plan as identified in the OSHA regulation for the Employee's Right to Know
   2. State the complete title for the acronym: MSDS
   3. Identify where the chemical manuals (MSDS) are located for the hospital as well as the department specific chemical manual.
   4. Identify the department specific chemicals that require spill kits and discuss the required procedure.

*(continued)*

C. Managing Risks
   1. Discuss the relationship of using safety procedures to reduce risks of injury or damage to patients, employees, visitors, medical staff, volunteers, students, and the facility property.
   2. Describe the procedure to follow when an injury or damage occurs.
   3. Discuss the documentation procedures to follow to report an injury or damage (incident report) and identify the process used for investigation of each incident.
   4. Identify the most common injuries in a hospital and discuss what corrective action has occurred to reduce the risk.
D. Using Employee Health Services When Ill or Injured
   1. Identify illnesses or injury that are reported to employee health.
   2. Discuss the method used to receive Worker's Compensation if injured on the job.
   3. Describe procedures used by Employee Health to reduce illness exposure to employee by use of an Infection Control Plan.
E. Establishing a Back Safety Program for Employees
   1. List the rules for "Good Body Mechanics"
   2. Demonstrate lifting techniques (used to reduce injury)
   3. Identify the rules necessary for transporting or moving patients safely to reduce injury to the patient and the employee.

**F–3**

## SAFETY TRAINING PROGRAM POSTTEST

Name _____  Date _____

*Directions: Utilizing information presented in the safety training program, answer the following questions in a clear and concise fashion.*

1. Identify code names for the following conditions:

   Fire _____

   Cardiac arrest _____

   Disruptive behavior _____

2. Define the meaning of the acronym RACE in the fire safety plan and describe the steps for how it is used.

   R _____

   _____

   A _____

   _____

   C _____

   _____

   E _____

   _____

3. The chemical manual for the diagnostic imaging department is

   located _____.

4. a) Name a chemical utilized in the department which requires a spill kit and b) explain the procedure to follow when that chemical is spilled.

   a. _____

   b._____

*(continued)*

_____

_____

5. List three (3) safety measures that will reduce the risks of injury or damage to patients, equipment or staff.

_____

_____

_____

6. Briefly describe the procedure to follow when a patient injury occurs.

_____

_____

_____

7. List three (3) illnesses or injuries which must be reported to employee health.

_____

_____

_____

8. List four (4) rules for "Good Body Mechanics."

_____

_____

_____

_____

## TAYLOR COUNTY HOSPITAL
## DEPARTMENT OF EDUCATIONAL SERVICES
## COMPETENCY/CREDENTIALING
## JOB TITLE: EDUCATOR

NAME: _____ DATE: _____

SSN: _____ DEPARTMENT: _____

### EVALUATION CODE:

**NOVICE:** Satisfactory—An average employee whose performance is sufficient to consider that the requirements of the position are being met. Generally performed at minimal level of established objectives with the results that overall contribution was marginal. Performance required an unusually high degree of supervision. (This level is considered acceptable only for employees new to the job.)

**APPRENTICE:** Needs Improvement—An average employee whose performance, while not being unsatisfactory, cannot be considered fully proficient. Generally met established objectives and expectations but definite areas exist where achievement needs improvement. Performance required somewhat more than normal degree of direction and supervision.

**PROFICIENT:** Meets Expectations—A fully acceptable employee who consistently meets all requirements of position accountabilities. Has consistently met established objectives in a satisfactory and adequate manner. Performance required normal degree of supervision and direction. (This level of performance should apply to the majority of employees.)

**DISTINGUISHED:** Exceeds Expectations—An above-average employee whose performance is clearly above what is considered to be acceptable. Has usually performed beyond established objectives and, at times, has made contributions beyond responsibilities of present position. Requires less than normal expected degree of direction and supervision.

**EXPERT:** Far Exceeds Expectations—A truly outstanding employee whose achievements are far above what is considered to be acceptable. Has consistently performed far beyond established objectives and has made significant contributions beyond current position. Requires minimal direction and supervision. (Relatively few employees would normally be expected to achieve at this level.)

**F–4(b)**

## TAYLOR COUNTY HOSPITAL
## ORIENTATION/COMPETENCY ASSESSMENT

NAME: _____ JOB TITLE: _____

SKILL: _____

The employee will be able to:
1.
2.
3.
4.
5.

SELF ASSESSMENT:
DEFINITIONS: 1. Competence means "able to perform procedure safely, correctly, effectively, and legally."
2. Performance level competency terms are:
N - Novice
A - Apprentice
P - Proficient
D - Distinguished
E - Expert
DIRECTIONS: Initial the appropriate answer and/or note the correct performance level abbreviations for each of the following questions.

ACTION PLAN: The Instructor or Evaluator must initial the appropriate action

1. Learn/Teach: Gain knowledge through classroom and/or laboratory activity.
2. Practice: Reinforce learning with or without assistance.
3. Perform: Accomplish goal independently.

| DATE | HAVE YOU EVER PERFORMED THIS PROCEDURE? | | ARE YOU COMPETENT IN PERFORMING THIS PROCEDURE? | | BASED ON YOUR COMPETENCY PLEASE DESCRIBE YOUR PERFORMANCE LEVEL. | LEARN | PRACTICE | PERFORM |
|---|---|---|---|---|---|---|---|---|
| | YES | NO | YES | NO | | | | |
| | | | | | | | | |
| | | | | | | | | |
| | | | | | | | | |
| | | | | | | | | |
| | | | | | | | | |
| | | | | | | | | |
| | | | | | | | | |

| DATE | INITIAL | NAME | TITLE |
|---|---|---|---|
| | | | |
| | | | |
| | | | |

DEPARTMENT: _____ DATE OF HIRE: _____

VALIDATION/EVALUATION: The Evaluator must date and initial the appropriate validation category. Performance level competency terms are:

    N - Novice
    A - Apprentice
    P - Proficient
    D - Distinguished
    E - Expert

This is to certify that the above individual has demonstrated the ability to perform the technical/clerical skills listed in a simulated training environment, clinical or work setting or a verbal demonstration method within the guidelines of the skill criteria.

| SIMULATION OF TRAINING | | WORK SETTING OR CLINICAL | | VERBAL DEMONSTRATION | | PERFORMANCE LEVEL | COMMENTS |
|---|---|---|---|---|---|---|---|
| DATE | INITIAL | DATE | INITIAL | DATE | INITIAL | | |
| | | | | | | | |
| | | | | | | | |
| | | | | | | | |
| | | | | | | | |
| | | | | | | | |
| | | | | | | | |

| DATE | INITIAL | NAME | | TITLE |
|---|---|---|---|---|
| | | | | |
| | | | | |
| | | | | |

F–4(c)

## TAYLOR COUNTY HOSPITAL
## ORIENTATION/COMPETENCY ASSESSMENT

NAME: _____

SOCIAL SECURITY NUMBER: _____

DEPARTMENT: _Educational Services_____

JOB TITLE: _Director of Educational Services_____

DATE OF HIRE: _____

SELF ASSESSMENT:
DEFINITIONS: 1. Competence means "able to perform procedure safely, correctly, effectively, and legally."
2. Performance level competency terms are:
  N - Novice
  A - Apprentice
  P - Proficient
  D - Distinguished
  E - Expert
DIRECTIONS: Initial the appropriate answer and/or note the correct performance level abbreviations for each of the following questions.

ACTION PLAN: The Instructor or Evaluator must initial the appropriate action

1. Learn/Teach: Gain knowledge through classroom and/or laboratory activity.
2. Practice: Reinforce learning with or without assistance.
3. Perform: Accomplish goal independently.

| DATE | HAVE YOU EVER PERFORMED THIS PROCEDURE? | | ARE YOU COMPETENT IN PERFORMING THIS PROCEDURE? | | BASED ON YOUR COMPETENCY PLEASE DESCRIBE YOUR PERFORMANCE LEVEL. | LEARN | PRACTICE | PERFORM |
|---|---|---|---|---|---|---|---|---|
| | YES | NO | YES | NO | | | | |
| | | | | | | | | |
| | | | | | | | | |
| | | | | | | | | |
| | | | | | | | | |
| | | | | | | | | |
| | | | | | | | | |

| DATE | INITIAL | NAME | TITLE |
|---|---|---|---|
| | | | |
| | | | |
| | | | |

SKILL: <u>FIRE SAFETY</u>

The employee will be able to:

Criteria: <u>1. Review ADM. Policy 500-1 and 500-29</u>

        <u>2. Review Fire Emergency Plan</u>

        <u>3. Define the Acronym R.A.C.E.</u>

        <u>4. Locate main hospital emergency exits</u>

VALIDATION/EVALUATION: The Evaluator must date and initial the appropriate validation category. Performance level competency terms are:

    N - Novice
    A - Apprentice
    P - Proficient
    D - Distinguished
    E - Expert

This is to certify that the above individual has demonstrated the ability to perform the technical/clerical skills listed in a simulated training environment, clinical or work setting or a verbal demonstration method within the guidelines of the skill criteria.

| STIMULATION OF TRAINING | | WORK SETTING OR CLINICAL | | VERBAL DEMONSTRATION | | PERFORMANCE LEVEL | COMMENTS |
|---|---|---|---|---|---|---|---|
| DATE | INITIAL | DATE | INITIAL | DATE | INITIAL | | |
| | | | | | | | |
| | | | | | | | |
| | | | | | | | |
| | | | | | | | |
| | | | | | | | |
| | | | | | | | |

| DATE | INITIAL | NAME | | TITLE |
|---|---|---|---|---|
| | | | | |
| | | | | |
| | | | | |

F–5

---

## CLINICAL SKILL ANALYSIS

NAME ⎯⎯⎯⎯⎯⎯⎯⎯⎯⎯⎯⎯

**Procedure** ⎯⎯⎯⎯⎯⎯⎯⎯⎯⎯⎯⎯⎯⎯⎯⎯⎯⎯⎯⎯⎯⎯

If the employee performs the specific skill circle yes (Y); if the skill is not performed circle no (N).

The employee:

| | | | | | |
|---|---|---|---|---|---|
| evaluated the requisition | Y N | | | | |
| identified the appropriate patient (100%) | Y N | | | | |
| asked and received pertinent history (98%) | Y N | | | | |
| assessed patient/explained procedure (98%) | Y N | | | | |
| prepared the room (95%) | Y N | | | | |

| **Position** | ⎯⎯ | ⎯⎯ | ⎯⎯ |
|---|---|---|---|
| selected appropriate film size | Y N | Y N | Y N |
| positioned anatomy correctly | Y N | Y N | Y N |
| appropriately positioned central ray | Y N | Y N | Y N |
| collimated to the anatomy | Y N | Y N | Y N |
| gave appropriate directions to patient | Y N | Y N | Y N |
| selected correct exposure factors | Y N | Y N | Y N |
| used appropriate radiation protection | Y N | Y N | Y N |
| film was appropriately marked (R or L) | Y N | Y N | Y N |
| correct anatomy was displayed | Y N | Y N | Y N |
| finished radiograph of good diagnostic quality | Y N | Y N | Y N |

The employee:   completed ⎯⎯⎯ remediation ⎯⎯⎯ retest ⎯⎯⎯

Comments: ⎯⎯⎯⎯⎯⎯⎯⎯⎯⎯⎯⎯⎯⎯⎯⎯⎯⎯⎯⎯

**Signatures:**

⎯⎯⎯⎯⎯⎯⎯⎯⎯⎯⎯⎯     ⎯⎯⎯⎯⎯⎯⎯⎯⎯⎯

Evaluator                              Date

⎯⎯⎯⎯⎯⎯⎯⎯⎯⎯⎯⎯

Employee

# Professional Organizations and State Agencies

## ACCREDITING AGENCIES

Joint Review Committee on Education in Diagnostic Medical Sonography
7108-C South Alton Way
Englewood, CO 80112-2106
(303) 741-3533

Joint Review Committee on Education in Radiologic Technology
20 North Wacker Drive, Suite 900
Chicago, IL 60606-2901
(312) 704-5300

Joint Review Committee on Educational Programs in Nuclear Medicine
   Technology
1144 West 3300 South
Salt Lake City, UT 84119
(801) 975-1144

## CERTIFICATION AGENCIES

American Registry of Diagnostic Medical Sonographers
2368 Victory Parkway, Suite 510
Cincinnati, OH 45206
(800) 541-9754
(513) 281-7111

American Registry of Radiologic Technologists
1255 Northland Drive
St. Paul, MN 55120-1155
(612) 687-0048

Nuclear Medicine Technology Certification Board
2970 Clairmont Road NE, Suite 610
Atlanta, GA 30329-1634
(404) 315-1739

# PROFESSIONAL SOCIETIES

American Healthcare Radiology Administrators
111 Boston Post Road, Suite 215
PO Box 334
Sudbury, MA 01766
(508) 443-7591

American Society of Radiologic Technologists
15000 Central Avenue SE
Albuquerque, NM 87123-3909
(505) 298-4500

Association of Educators in the Radiologic Sciences
2021 Spring Road, Suite 600
Oak Brook, IL 60521
(708) 571-9183

International Society of Radiographers and Radiologic Technologists
ISRRT Secretary-General
52 Addison Crescent
Don Mills, Ontario M3B 1K8
Canada

Society of Diagnostic Medical Sonographers
12225 Greenville Ave., Suite 434
Dallas, TX 75243
(214) 235-7367

Society for Magnetic Resonance Imaging
1918 University Ave., Suite C
Berkeley, CA 94704
(510) 841-1899

Society of Nuclear Medicine—Technologist Section
136 Madison Avenue
New York, NY 10016-6784
(212) 889-0717

## OTHER ORGANIZATIONS

American Association of Physicists in Medicine
335 East 45th St.
New York, NY 10017
(212) 661-9404

American Board of Radiology
2301 West Big Beaver Rd., Suite 625
Troy, MI 48084
(313) 643-0300

American College of Radiology
1891 Preston White Drive
Reston, VA 22091
(703) 648-8900

American Institute of Ultrasound in Medicine
11200 Rockville Pike, Suite 205
Rockville, MD 20852-3139
(301) 881-2486

American Society of Therapeutic Radiology and Oncology
1101 Market Street, Suite 1400
Philadelphia, PA 19107
(215) 574-3185

Radiological Society of North America
2021 Spring Road, Suite 600
Oak Brook, IL 60521
(708) 571-2670

## STATE LICENSING AGENCIES

Arizona
  State of Arizona
  Medical Radiologic Technology Board of Examiners
  4814 South 40th St.
  Phoenix, AZ 85040
  (602) 255-4845

California
  State of California
  Radiologic Health Branch
  714 P Street
  Sacramento, CA 95814
  (916) 445-6695

Delaware
  State of Delaware
  Office of Radiation Control
  Robbins Bldg.
  PO Box 637
  Dover, DE 19903
  (302) 736-4731

Florida
  State of Florida
  Radiologic Health Program
  1317 Winewood Blvd.
  Tallahassee, FL 32399-0700
  (904) 487-3451

Hawaii
  State of Hawaii
  Radiologic Technology Board
  Department of Health
  Noise and Radiation Branch
  591 Ala Moana Blvd.
  Honolulu, HI 96813-2498
  (808) 548-4383

Illinois
  State of Illinois
  Division of Radiologic Technologist Certification
  Illinois Department of Nuclear Safety
  1035 Outer Park Dr.
  Springfield, IL 62704
  (217) 785-9915

Indiana
  State of Indiana
  Radiological Health Section
  PO Box 1964
  Indianapolis, IN 46206-1964
  (317) 633-0150

Iowa
  State of Iowa
  Department of Health
  Lucas State Office Bldg.
  Des Moines, IA 50319-0075
  (515) 281-3478

Kentucky
  State of Kentucky
  Radiation Control Branch
  275 East Main Street
  Frankfort, KY 40621
  (502) 564-3700

Louisiana
  Louisiana State Radiologic Technology Board of Examiners
  3108 Cleary Ave., Suite 207
  Metairie, LA 70002
  (504) 838-5231

Maine
  State of Maine
  Radiologic Technology Board of Examiners
  State House Station #35
  Augusta, ME 04333
  (207) 582-8723

Maryland
  State of Maryland
  Public Health Engineer
  2500 Broening Highway
  Baltimore, MD 21224
  (301) 631-3300

Massachusetts
  State of Massachusetts
  Radiation Control Program
  150 Tremont Street, 11th Floor
  Boston, MA 02111
  (617) 727-6214

Montana
  State of Montana
  Department of Commerce
  Board of Radiologic Technologists
  1424 Ninth Avenue
  Helena, MT 59620
  (406) 444-4288

Nebraska
  State of Nebraska
  Division of Radiological Health
  301 Centennial Mall South
  Lincoln, NE 68509
  (402) 471-2168

New Jersey
  State of New Jersey
  Department of Environmental Protection
  Bureau of Radiological Health
  CN 415
  Trenton, NJ 08625-0415
  (609) 987-2022

New Mexico
  State of New Mexico
  Radiation Protection Bureau
  PO Box 968
  Santa Fe, NM 87504-0968
  (505) 827-2773 or (505) 827-2941

New York
  Bureau of Environment Radiation Protection
  New York State Department of Health, Rm. 325
  2 University Place
  Albany, NY 12203
  (518) 458-6482

Oregon
  Health Licensing Boards
  Oregon State Health Division
  PO Box 231
  Portland, OR 97207
  (503) 229-5054

Tennessee
  State of Tennessee
  Board of Medical Examiners
  283 Plus Park Blvd.
  Nashville, TN 37217
  (615) 367-6231
Texas
  Texas Department of Health
  Medical Radiologic Technology Program
  1100 West 49th St.
  Austin, TX 78756-3183
  (512) 459-2960
Vermont
  State of Vermont
  Board of Radiologic Technology
  Division of Licensing and Registration
  Pavilion Office Bldg.
  Montpelier, VT 05609-1101
  (802) 828-2886
Washington
  Washington State Office of Radiation
  Olympic Bldg.   Suite 220
  217 Pine Street
  Seattle, WA 98101-1549
  (206) 464-6840
West Virginia
  State of West Virginia
  Valley One Complex, Room 303
  3049 Robert C. Byrd Dr.
  Beckley, WV 25801
  (304) 256-6985
Wyoming
  State of Wyoming
  Board of Radiologic Technologist Examiners
  1312 Monroe Avenue
  Cheyenne, WY 82001
  (307) 778-7319
Puerto Rico
  University of Puerto Rico
  Medical Science Campus
  Department of Environmental Health
  G.P.O. Box 5067
  San Juan, PR 00936
  (809) 758-2525 ext. 1424

# I N D E X

Note: Page numbers in italics refer to sample forms.

ISBN 0-7216-5062-7

90038

9 780721 650623